# Natural Remedies

## Ultimate Guide For Using Plants &Herbs To Heal Your Body & Mind

*(Herbal Medicine For Common Ailments And For Cleaning, Beauty, And Wellness)*

**Robert Zion**

Published By **Chris David**

# Robert Zion

*Natural Remedies: Ultimate Guide For Using Plants & Herbs To Heal Your Body & Mind (Herbal Medicine For Common Ailments And For Cleaning, Beauty, And Wellness)*

**ISBN   978-1-77485-972-8**

No part of this guidebook shall be reproduced in any form without permission in writing from the publisher except in the case of brief quotations embodied in critical articles or reviews.

Legal & Disclaimer

# Table of Contents

## Chapter 1: Natural Herbal Remedies: An Introduction

I am glad you decided to take this journey with us and I hope you find exactly what you need. I'd like to briefly explain the reasons I created this book. This book is meant for you to get the most information possible. If you feel that the text gives too much detail, don't worry! That is the way it was created so that you can get the most from it. Let's get started! !

What is it that natural remedies can do for you? Many people are not aware of the many benefits that natural remedies offer. They are more comfortable taking prescribed medications or ones they are already familiar with. This is fine. However, it is important to consider the possible side effects that these chemicals can cause. Because these remedies are natural, many people resort to natural remedies for their ailments. You can find herbs, vegetables, and fruits in many of these remedies. The best thing is that many of these items can be found in every kitchen.

But can it really work? The answer is yes, considering that natural medicines have been used throughout history. This was before modern medicine was created and synthetic drugs became popular. It works. However, how effective it is depends on the individual. However, doctors often recommend using them instead of relying on prescription medicine for simple ailments. Some illnesses can be cured even by eating healthy foods. It would be a good idea to harness these healing properties and make them available as supplements to medications. It is possible to use the natural remedy by itself if it is powerful enough. Studies and research show that many natural remedies work the same way as synthetic medications.

How can you get started? First of all, you'll need to be familiar with the ingredients needed to treat a specific condition. This is where this book will come in handy. We'll discuss the details more later.

Fresh food, herbs, and spices can all be used effectively to treat most ailments. These can range from minor discomforts to serious infections. Antibiotics are often used to treat such ailments. Let's be real, antibiotics can be costly and can sometimes cause serious side effects if they are not used properly. Also, antibiotics can cause harm to beneficial flora/fauna in our bodies. This makes recovery time longer. In the worst cases, they could backfire and damage our immune systems. You can avoid it all with natural home remedies. It not only treats the actual problem, but it also strengthens your immune system so it is better equipped to fight off other illnesses. It also helps to heal various aches and hurts.

Other than medicine, home remedies can be used to make your mouthwash or toothpaste. Some people go as far as creating their own medicinal soaps, which allow them to avoid the mass-marketed products that could contain ingredients that are harmful to the skin or don't support the skin.

While it is more difficult to make these soaps, a few hours should suffice if the effort is worthwhile. For those with skin issues, the instructions for making natural soap are in the next chapters. Consider making your own remedies for constipation. This would work well if you require regular food to allow your bowel to move easily.

These home remedies may also be useful for other reasons. There are also home remedies that you can use to help your loved one or yourself recover faster from the flu. You can make teas to help with a sore throat, a cough, or other symptoms. A throat spray is a common treatment for asthma. Natural ingredients are much more affordable than store-bought ones.

Although we've mentioned it before, these remedies are not only meant to be used internally. In addition to the mouthwash and soaps, it is possible to make your own natural cleansers that treat skin conditions such a acne. Natural ingredients can also be used to make an antiseptic spray. This is useful for treating dermatitis. It can also help heal blisters.

It is clear that there are many things one can do in home remedies. The only thing you really need is a guideline and some time to do research. You'll be more comfortable mixing recipes and learning about the benefits associated with a particular ingredient.

## Chapter 2: Hair Loss Effects

Why is it so important that we act on hair loss as soon as possible? Good hair habits are essential to avoid this happening. If you have already been diagnosed with the condition, natural remedies can help.

Hair loss can have different effects depending on how one feels about it. While some people can resume their daily routines after hair loss occurs, others become more anxious, shy, or stressed.

Here are some common symptoms of hair loss that affect people who are affected emotionally by the condition.

1. Sometimes, people become frustrated when they are unable to style their hair in the way that they desire. Some people find it difficult to do hairstyles that conceal their problem.

2. Many people feel older and feel less desirable.

3. People become lonely looking in the mirror. This causes them to be unhappy and disturbed.

4. Low self-esteem is often a result of being less confident in your appearance. Emotionally, the

condition can cause you to withdraw from people you used be able to interact with. If you do not stop, it could lead to a reduced social circle and a lonely lifestyle.

5. It can be hard for those who are so picky about their hair to admit that they are losing their hair. This can be very distressing especially when you realize you cannot do the same hair care routines as you used to.

6. Women and men who lose their hair feel embarrassed and lack confidence. Males tend to avoid the other sex. Women are more insecure than men and will continue to seek out ways to hide their condition.

7. If the condition becomes more obvious, people tend to get concerned about being teased and humiliated. Studies have shown that at least 50% of bald people have experienced being teased or humiliated about their condition.

8. This can cause a person to lose their effectiveness at work, particularly if they are constantly in front cameras or have to interact with a lot.

While hair loss can be a serious problem, it is possible to make positive changes to your outlook.

These are some of these things you can do that will boost your self-confidence and help you maintain your self-esteem, even if your hair is falling out.

1. Other reasons to compliment people are plenty. You might lose your hair but you can be nicer and more confident. Try to make it seem like your hair is fine and that you aren't bothered by it.

2. Why fret about hair loss when your focus should be on getting a better body shape? To make yourself fitter and healthier, you can also start a daily fitness routine.

3. Think about the numerous studies done on baldmen when you feel low. Many people perceived bald men to be more intelligent, successful, assertive than their peers.

If you are unable to do anything about the problem then your best friend is your self-confidence and self-esteem. Keep these two things in your heart. These two things will help you to deal with the fact of your hair being thinner. You can also get your outlook back on track.

## Chapter 3: Beauty That Shines With Essential Oils

Essential oils have been a beauty favorite for decades. They are often used in moisturizers for their moisturizing, soothing and rich properties. Here are some examples of essential oils used today and in the past to help you achieve natural and radiant beauty.

1) Sunflower Oil

Sunflower oil is extracted from sunflower seed oils, which are rich sources of Vitamin E.

a. Reduces the appearance of scarring or other marks.

b. Moisturize the face, hair, and nails

c. Use to moisturize the eyes and reduce puffiness.

d. Treats skin irritations and insect bites

e. Act as an overall body moisturizer that is gentle enough for those with sensitive skin

f. Serves as a makeup remover

These are just a few of the many benefits that this miracle oil offers. You won't regret buying at least one bottle. It is easy to find sunflower oil, as well as its by-products, on the market.

2) Baobab Oil

Baobab Oil can be described as an essential oil derived directly from the seeds the Baobab tree. Although the Baobab tree is sometimes found in other countries, it is indigenous to Africa. This oil was first used to treat muscle aches in Africa. This oil has many other uses. People from Zambia used this oil for bathing babies. It became a beauty staple, used to maintain skin elasticity, regeneration and to keep a beautiful complexion.

Camellia Oil

You need healthy hair to achieve that ageless beauty. Don't forget your hair! Hair is the crowning glory that can make or ruin your appearance. Now, the question is: How can you maintain healthy hair? Camellia Oil may be able to help!

Camellia Oil can be used by Japanese women to keep their hair shiny and healthy. Camellia Oil's high oleic and protein content makes it perfect for nourishment. Camellia Oil is powerful enough to eliminate the need for hot oil treatment. Simply apply a teaspoonful of Camellia Oil on your hair and wrap it with a towel for 20-30 mins.

4) Tea Tree Oil

People have a lot of facial problems nowadays, including blemishes and pimples. People find it difficult to keep their face clean and smooth due to all the dirt that surrounds them.

Tea Tree Oil is a common remedy for the same problem. Tea Tree Oil has anti-oxidant and cleansing properties which help reduce the appearance of acne. It is also high in vitamins to keep your skin healthy and beautiful.

5) Chamomile Oil

Stress is one of many major causes of premature ageing. It is inevitable but there are still ways to ease stress and keep your skin looking great. Aromatherapy, which Chamomile Oil is undoubtedly the best partner for this purpose, is one of the oldest ways to do it.

Chamomile Oil's relaxing scent can help ease tension in your body and mind. It has moisturizing properties, which can keep your skin moisturized and fresh. Drop a few drops into your bathtub to relax and moisturize your skin.

These oils are essential to a radiant, younger-looking you. These oils have no chemical additives, and are safer than commercial moisturizers. Keep in mind that your skin deserves the very best.

## Chapter 4: Dealing Avec Anxiety

Anxiety and insomnia can both lead to insomnia. Sleepless nights can even worsen anxiety. You think less about falling asleep and the more problems you have falling asleep. It's a vicious circle. You fear you'll be tossing around all night, so you begin to dread going back to bed. The fact that there is a huge project or presentation at school the next day may cause you to stress. If you don't have a restful night, you could be unable to pass a test. You are only increasing the problem by constantly thinking about your sleep problems and expecting that insomnia will hit when you go to bed. The more you dwell on the fact that you might have difficulty falling asleep, the greater your body's production of adrenaline. The more adrenaline in your body, you feel more awake.

Your thoughts regarding sleep and bedtime need to be reprogrammed. Rewire your brain to think about sleeping in your bedroom. If you put yourself in a bad mood, you might have difficulty falling asleep. Your anxiety about falling sleep may be keeping you from unwinding and relaxing before bedtime. You can retrain your brain to associate sleep with your bed.

Only use your bedroom to sleep. Don't bring work to bed. Avoid watching television or using electronic devices, such as your tablet, smartphone, or computer, in bed. It is important to associate your bed only with sleeping, so that when you go to bed, it is time for you to go to sleep.

You may have difficulty falling asleep. Instead of turning your head all night, get up and move around. Do not force yourself into sleeping. As you get more anxious, you'll be more likely to toss and turn. Get up and move out of your bedroom. Do something calm and relaxing. Read a good book. Make a cup if herbal, caffeine-free coffee. You can take a hot bath. You can listen to soothing or classical music. If you feel tired, turn on some soothing music and go back to bed.

You can move your clock to the side if you feel anxious while lying in bed. You will be more disturbed if your clock keeps ticking away while you try to fall asleep. Watching the clock constantly to find out the hours until your alarm rings will only cause you to be more stressed by the next morning. The alarm clock is still available; however, it should not be visible from any place.

You shouldn't have unrealistic expectations of yourself when you fall asleep. It is possible to have a great night's sleep by changing how you think.

Examples of positive self-talk

It is not true that everyone can fall asleep.

Instead, try this: Everyone experiences difficulty falling asleep at least once in their lifetime. This is completely normal and I'll overcome it.

It is not a good idea to say "This is another night without sleep." It is the exact same as every other night.

Instead, try this: Some nights I'm more able to fall asleep faster than others.

It is not true that I say "If I don't fall asleep, my job will be lost or I will fail my test."

Instead, tell yourself: I will complete my presentation or pass the big exam. I will make every effort to relax so that tomorrow is a great day.

It is not possible to say, "This cannot be done." I will never be capable of falling asleep. Everything is out my control.

Instead, think: I won't worry if I fall asleep. Worrying will only keep me awake more. I can conquer insomnia if I keep my mind positive.

It is not a good idea to say: "It will take me at least two hours to get to sleep."

Instead, use the following: I don't know what the future holds. My past experience with difficulty falling asleep does not guarantee that I will be able to do it again tonight. If I apply the strategies I have learned, it is possible to fall asleep quickly tonight.

Changes in your mind about sleep will take time. It is important to be patient. You can keep practicing these positive thoughts about falling asleep. All negative thoughts must be kept at bay.

## Chapter 5: Natural Remedies To Lower Blood Pressure

The use of natural remedies to treat and control aliments is not new. But it has experienced a significant increase in popularity over the past few years. This may be due to the convenience of accessing information online, as well as the fact that many people want a safer way of managing their health. There are natural remedies for hypertension.

Drink Hibiscus Tea

People all over the world have used hibiscus to lower blood pressure. Studies showed that hibiscus acts naturally as a diuretic. It will draw sodium from your bloodstream. This lowers blood pressure. Hibiscus seems to mimic ACE inhibitions, which are common prescription drugs for high blood pressure. While hibiscus might not be as potent than prescription ACE medicines, it can be very effective.

You will need these ingredients to make hibiscus ice tea:

* 1 to 2 teaspoons dried Hibiscus

* About 1 cup hot water

* Lemon, honey, 1 ½  to 2 cinnamon stiks (optional).

Bring the water to boil in a large pot. Allow the water to boil for five to eight minutes. If you're using cinnamon sticks, add them. To taste, stir in the honey. You can drink the tea up to three times a day.

Coconut Water

Coconut water is found inside the shell of unripe green coconuts. It contains magnesium and potassium that are crucial for healthy muscle function. We all know that the heart is a huge muscle. Although there is very little scientific evidence about the effects coconut water has on blood pressure and blood pressure, many people claim that coconut water can lower blood sugar when taken regularly. For this natural remedy, you can drink 8 ounces (8 to 2 per day) of coconut water. You can have the water both morning and night if you are able.

Take fish oil

Fish oil is everywhere, and it's a great supplement. It is. Omega-3 fatty oils are an important part of heart health. Experts agree that fish oil can reduce blood pressure. Many heart transplant patients have received fish oil to help lower their risk of hypertension after the procedure.

Eat Melon Every Morning

Watermelon isn't just a summer favorite, it can also lower blood tension. Citrulline, an essential amino acid, is found in watermelon. This organic compound will be converted into L-arginine by the body when it is consumed. Nitric oxide is also a precursor. Nitric oxide also regulates the flow of blood through the body. Nitric oxide can also increase blood vessel size, which reduces blood pressure. You only need to eat watermelon each morning on an empty stomach in order to reap these health benefits.

## Chapter 6: Natural Remedies Against Constipation

There are few things worse than feeling constipated. Bloating, fullness, a tight stomach, and uncomfortable feeling is what makes it so miserable. These natural remedies can relieve constipation and help you identify triggers.

Oil

Oils such as olive and coconut oils can be used for more than just cooking. They can also relieve constipation symptoms. Oils are rich in healthy fats which encourage digestion. They also help keep your digestive tract lubricated, allowing you to move food smoothly. These healthy fats can be found in avocados.

Lemon Juice

The celebrity cleansing diets that you have heard so much about are true. Although all remedies may not be the same, the citric acid found in lemons can help restore your digestive system. Lemon water can have a powerful effect on your digestive tract if taken before breakfast. Mix eight ounces warm water with one lemon juice. This breakfast lemonade will instantly awaken your sleepy stomach and restore regularity to your life.

Hydration

64 ounces is the recommended water intake for the average person. You will notice a decrease in your digestive speed if you drink less water. The slower your food is processed, the less water you ingest. This is because your body has fewer fluids. Therefore, constipation. Drinking water more will aid in flushing out toxins.

Caffeine

We all know that caffeine can be a stimulant. This makes it easy to see how it could help with your digestion. Caffeine, in particular, can also be a diuretic. Too much coffee can dehydrate you and make your constipation worse or worsen. You can start with one cup of black coffee after drinking lemon water in the morning. Keep going until you see the results. Take a few glasses of water and, if that doesn't work, have another cup.

Exercise

Get moving! This is a great way for your digestive system to be active. An exercise routine is an excellent motivator to speed up a slow digestive system. Sitting is a major part of our daily lives, so it's important to make an effort and get up the stairs. It's amazing for digestion and is often listed in the list of benefits to yoga. All the twisting, bending and turning can help to'massage your internal organs' and kick your digestive system into high speed. YouTube even has yoga lessons that focus on digestive health. Give it a go and see the results!

Fiber

Many foods you see in grocery stores boast 'added fiber'. There are two types: soluble or insoluble fiber. Both have their advantages. Soluble fibre is what makes you feel full because it forms gels to slow down digestion. Soluble fiber slows down stomach emptying, which aids in controlling blood sugar levels. Good for insulin health, but not great for constipation. Some foods that contain soluble fiber are:

* Oatmeal

* Apples

* Lentils

* Pears

* Flaxseeds

* Blueberries

Insoluble fiber is the answer to constipation. Insoluble fiber acts as a laxative, since it does not absorb any water. It passes through your body intact, which speeds up food's digestion. These foods can contain insoluble fibre:

* Nuts

* Whole grains

* Brown rice

* Zucchini

* Cucumbers

* Tomatoes

* Dark, leafy green vegetables

* Grapes & raisins

* Root vegetables

Constipation can often be alleviated by drinking plenty of water and insoluble fiber-rich food. The Dietary Guidelines for Americans 2010 found that Americans consume just 15g of fiber each day. This is close to half of what they should be eating. The recommendation for fiber is approximately 14 grams per 1,000 calories. For women, this equates to about 25 grams and for men, it is around 38 grams.

Bacteria

There are good bacteria and bad bacteria. Bad bacteria can make people more susceptible to getting sick. But good bacteria will keep them healthy. It is crucial to keep your digestive tract in tip-top shape by maintaining healthy stomach bacteria. This is particularly true considering the abundance of processed foods, added sugars, and other unhealthy food choices in today's American diet.

There are many methods to improve and maintain healthy stomach flora. This will help relieve and prevent constipation. Your body will stay healthy and strong by including yogurt that contains live cultures (the label will tell you this). A pill form of probiotics is another way to keep your stomach healthy and active. The proper balance of stomach bacteria will allow your body to absorb more nutrients.

## Chapter 7: Natural Remedies - Seasonal Ailments

Many ailments can be caused by changes in the weather. This is not surprising as your body has to adjust to changing weather conditions. Your body attempts to stay cool when it's hot in the summer. Your body will work harder to keep warm when it is winter. Your body has to fight off allergens in the spring.

Summer Ailments

Summer is the best month to hit the beaches, but summer also brings the most sunburns. Aloe Vera gel is a great option to prevent sunburns. To extract the gel, simply break open an Aloe Vera plant leaf. The gel should be applied directly to the area at least twice daily. Lavender oil is also an option to reduce scarring and speed-up healing.

The risk of developing athlete's toe is increased by heat, sweat and heat. Barefoot walking can increase the likelihood of having itchy, cracked and dry skin. Tea tree oil can be used as a natural remedy for athlete's heel. Tea tree oil has antifungal and healing properties. Use one-fourth of a teaspoon of olive oil, almond oil, or olive oil to combine several drops of teatree oil. The mixture can be used to rub your feet twice daily. You will notice a decrease in itching after several days. However you need to keep applying the mixture every day to your feet until the fungus disappears completely.

Summer is when bugs and ticks are most common. To relieve itching and swelling caused by bug bites, you can apply Echinacea oil directly to the affected area. To avoid infection, you can also put a few drops under your tongue. After you go outside, make it a habit to take a shower. You should inspect your skin for ticks. If you find any, take them off.

Winter Ailments

Your body adapts to temperature changes, climate changes, and diet in winter. Your body becomes more susceptible to infections and viruses as a result. Your body becomes more susceptible to infections such as cold, sore throat and cough. Additional symptoms that are common at this time include dry and itchy skin and congestion in the chest, nasal runniness, seasonal allergies and chest congestion. Allergy sufferers and those with arthritis can experience severe symptoms.

Tea tree oil has natural expectorant properties that can help with cold symptoms, such as congestion, cough, and bronchitis. Apply a small amount to your chest or on your pillow and inhale when you go to sleep. You can also use it to treat bronchitis or upper respiratory infections like cough or bronchitis. Make thyme tea by boiling two teaspoons of crushed leaves and one cup of water. Then cover the cup with a lid and let it steep for approximately ten minutes.

To treat dry cough, turmeric tea can be taken. Combine carom seeds with turmeric powder and boil water. To increase its healing powers, you can also add honey. Honey can be mildly antibiotic. Black pepper tea can be used to treat wet or mucusy cough. Mix honey and ground black pepper together in a cup. Leave it to boil for 15 minutes, then strain. Cayenne is an alternative if black pepper is unavailable. Natural oils like jojoba, coconut and avocado can be used for chapped and cracked skin.

Spring Ailments

Due to the seasonal changes in weather and the presence pollen in the atmosphere, seasonal allergies can occur in spring. Hay fever (also known as allergic rhinoitis) is quite common during spring. While not life-threatening, it can be a serious problem that can impact your daily activities. Start treatment immediately if you start to notice symptoms like watery eyes or sneezing, coughing, dry eyes, headaches, sinus congestion, and itchiness in your eyes, nose, throat and mouth.

To alleviate congestion and allergens, you could use a salicylic solution. Simply combine one-fourth of a teaspoon of salt with two cups (or more) of water in a squeeze container or netipot. Hay fever can also be treated by ginger mixed with honey and lime. The same goes for nettle extracts. The steam from inhaling can also help soothe your nasal passages. Simply add a few drops oil of peppermint or lavender to hot water, and inhale their steam.

Bayberry decoctions are a great way to boost your immune systems. Drinking green tea with high levels of antioxidants is also an option. Peppermint or chamomile tea can be used to treat any respiratory issues. Apple cider vinegar, reishi, turmeric and licorice root are all home remedies that you can use to treat seasonal allergic reactions. Goldenrod and elderflower are also recommended by the Herbal Academy of New England for seasonal allergies.

## Chapter 8: Gastrointestinal Remedies

Diarrhoea

Diarrhoea is a condition that can lead to serious health problems. The following can be used to treat diarrhoea.

* Fenugreek beans. Fenugreek's fibre content can help thicken the stool. Take half a teaspoon of Fenugreek seeds and add it to a glass of chilled water. Take three servings daily.

* Chamomile tea. Chamomile tea has natural properties that reduce inflammation in the intestinal tract. The Heartburn section has the recipe of the chamomile-chamomile Tea.

* Orange peel tea. The rind from oranges is an effective treatment for diarrhoea. This helps improve digestion and eliminates the bad bacteria that can cause diarrhoea. You can simply peel the entire orange and then mix it with 2 cups water. After that, let it sit for a while or until it is lukewarm.

* Salty and sweet drink. Take half a teaspoonful of salt and half a teaspoonful of sugar, and mix it

in a glass water. Repeat the process several times a days. You will be hydrated, but this solution can also help restore electrolytes from your body.

* Yoghurt. Yoghurt aids in the growth of good bacteria in your colon. This can help to stop diarrhoea. Three cups of yoghurt should be consumed daily, with natural yogurts and without any flavourings.

Constipation

Constipation is similar to diarrhoea. It can also be a hassle and cause for great pain. Sometimes it can cause even more serious complications. These natural remedies can help with constipation.

* Olive oil. Because oils are natural lubricants, they can help constipation. They can help ease the digestion process. Olive oil is not the best remedy for constipation, but you can combine it with some juice. Simply mix a tablespoon EVOO with half a cup of lemon juice or a full glass of lemon.

* Flax oil. Flax seed oils are effective in constipation, much like EVOO. Flax seed oil is easy

to take with lemon juice, orange juice, or the same as olive oils.

* Prunes. Prunes and prune juice are popular ways to get rid of constipation. They not only have a lot of fibre but also contain sorbitol (a substance which can soften the stool). Two glasses of wine per day is recommended, one each morning and one at dinner.

* Lemon. Citric acid, which is high in lemon, acts as a stimulant to your digestive system. It is also good for your colon and helps eliminate toxins. You can simply add fresh lemon to a cup full of warm water. In just a few moments, you can feel the results.

* Dandelion tea. The benefits of dandelion tea include natural laxatives and antioxidants. See the section on Joint Pain to learn how to make dandelion tee.

Bloating & Gas

Flatulence or bloating is not considered a serious condition, except for the rare instances when you accidentally release gas. These things are embarrassing and should not be taken lightly.

* Caraway seeds. Caraway seeds can be used to pass gas. If you feel bloated or can't expel the gas, caraway seeds are a good option.

* Anise seeds. Like caraway seeds, anise is a potent carminative that can help you let go of gas. It also contains anti-spasmodic compounds. You can also take a small amount of anise seeds to pass gas.

* Ginger. Yes, ginger. Because of the two compounds in ginger, shogaols as well as gingerol, ginger is a great carminative. They help reduce inflammation and relax colon. You can either chew small pieces throughout your day or consume a teaspoon of grated ginger prior to eating. Ginger tea can also be enjoyed (recipe for ginger-tea can be found under Headaches).

* Peppermint Tea. You'll see peppermint again in the spotlight, just like ginger. The anti-spasmodic properties of peppermint, along with its soothing properties for nerves, make it less painful. For the tea, boil 1 cup of water and add 1 tablespoon of peppermint leaf. Let it steep for 15 minutes. Strain the mixture and heat it up.

* Pumpkin. A great way to reduce the amount of gas produced during digestion is pumpkin. A cup of pumpkin should be consumed with every meal. These can be eaten raw, mashed, steamed, and even as a dessert.

Nausea

A nausea attack can be both bothersome and frustrating. Even though nausea isn't serious, particularly if it is caused by gastrointestinal issues, it should still be treated as soon as possible. This is possible by:

* Inhale lemon extract. Nausea is eased by the citrusy scent of lemons. By inhaling the scent of a single lemon slice, you can get rid of that nauseating sensation. Keep doing this until you are relieved of the nausea.

* Eat bread. You can relieve nausea by eating bread.

* Take in ginger. Ginger has many medicinal properties, including the ability to relieve nausea caused by acid. You can take either a glass of ginger tea, or a ginger broth. You can also chew small pieces until the sensation goes away.

* Peppermint. Peppermint's cooling and pleasant scent has been found to be a powerful remedy for nausea. It can be enjoyed as a tea or used as an ointment. Apply a few drops of peppermint essential oil to your gums and it will do its job. For a stronger scent, you can also inhale this oil.

## Chapter 9: Remedies For Arthritis, Pain In The Joints, And Muscle Problems

Arthritis can be a serious condition in the elderly population of western countries. It can be caused by age, but there are two main forms. The first, called rheumatoid (an immune system disorder), can be treated by proper diet and good use of herbal supplements. Osteosis is the wear and tear effect on joints and bones. The beauty of nature is back, as the majority of herbs we'll be looking at in this chapter are very effective when it comes curing inflammation.

What are the symptoms then? They include gout or fibromyalgia. No matter the type of arthritis, the discomfort and fatigue are inevitable. The classic medicine will not help, but it will reduce the symptoms. Or you can try herbal medicine, which will be less expensive and provide relief. You can always refer back to modern medicine. However, it would not hurt to give the option of natural treatments a try at least for a week.

It is vital to act as soon as you can because arthritis is one of most common and most severe conditions. Here are some basic treatments for arthritis that are considered to be more effective than both modern medical guidelines and drugstore remedies.

The interesting thing about arthritis is that it can be referred to as a "general" condition. Because it can affect multiple parts of the body at once, arthritis medications are typically prescribed for many other conditions. Herbalism is not an exception. These remedies can be used for most muscle and joint conditions, including more complex ones like headaches. Be careful not to experiment with conditions that aren't listed in each recipe.

Cat's claw oil

It may sound strange. Cat's claw can be a very helpful herb to help with inflammation. It is also a tincture so you don't have to be an expert in herbalism. The tannins in this tincture act as acids and the healing alkaloids. It is vital that they reach your stomach. Otherwise, they will lose their effectiveness.

For maximum effectiveness, it is recommended that you mix six ounces of water with the tincture. This will allow the tincture to be diluted enough to reach your stomach. Mix that with one tablespoon fresh squeezed lemon juice. Add one teaspoon of vinegar to make it amazing.

Birch Bark Tea

It is unsurpassed in its ability to treat sudden pains in joints and indisposition. To activate the natural remedies of the birch's chemistry, you will only need one tablespoon of fresh grated Ginger. It will also give the tea a slightly sweeter, but still hot, flavor. To make the tea, you will need 2 cups of birch bark (about 3 grams) and 3 grams ginger. To make the tea, boil 300 grams of water. Then add the ingredients. Once the tea has reached a boiling point, add honey or stevia. Clove and cinnamon are also options. However, you must ensure they don't cause any stomach irritation.

Cayenne infused oil

What makes this remedy a good choice to treat arthritis? It can be used through the skin, which makes it one of the most effective herbal remedies for treating arthritis. It is especially helpful when you have to deal with inflammation, severe symptoms and inability move. Cayenne oil offers a far better alternative to other irritating products, such as capsaicin and creams. Cayenne oil is also an effective treatment for lower back pain, sciatica, general muscle disorders and more. It is also a good massage oil and can help with headache relief.

For the remedy to be effective, you'll need four tablespoons of cayenne pepper paste and one cup olive oil. It is that easy. Mix everything together in a bowl until the mixture is homogenous. You can add menthol crystals or peppermint to enhance the scent. However, it won't harm the physical properties.

We now need to go into more detail. First, the proportion of oil to pepper that you use will depend on the heat of the peppers and your skin's sensitivities. For ten days you should use it at a low heat. You can also use it up until two weeks at about one hundred degrees Fahrenheit. Combine the ingredients and stir until well combined. The mixture should be left for at the least one night. You can then store the mixture at room temperature.

Cayenne menthol salve

Cayenne again, right? It is a powerful tool that can be used to naturally fight disease. Cayenne salves provide instant relief for common pains in the bones and muscles, especially chronic pain. The menthol gives energy to the body, and improves blood circulation. It also helps to cool the pain and blocks the nerve signals. The strength of the menthol depends on how often you use it.

Cayenne can be irritating and you need to be careful. First, try a small amount on a tiny area of your skin and see how it reacts. If it doesn't react in a way that is normal, you can continue to use the product. This is not recommended if you're pregnant or have liver problems.

Let's get started. Ingredients: One cup coconut oil, four teaspoons of cayenne, four tablespoons more of emulsifying oil, four extra tablespoons worth of menthol crystals, thirty drops oil blend and two tablespoons more of menthol.

If the coconut remains solid, heat it up until it liquefies. You shouldn't heat it too much as this can cause damage to the coconut's properties. Then, stir in the cayenne pepper and combine it. Once this is done, you will need to keep the mixture in warm place where you can easily stir it every day. After seven to 10 days, you can stop steering the mixture. However, you must continue heating the coconut oil to prevent it becoming too solid. Give the powder time to settle, then pour it into a metal-free bowl. Melt the wax in the microwave before adding it. Combine the mixture with the wax. Add the menthol crystals to the mixture and stir until it is dissolved. To increase the effect, you could add twenty drops to peppermint oils.

And that's it! It's a complex, but effective, remedy for swollen and irritated joints.

## Chapter 10: Hair Care Do's/Don'ts

It is important to understand what good and bad hair care habits are for your hair.

These are the "Do's" when it comes to hair care.

1. Keep in mind that your hair is very vulnerable when it's wet. Use a towel to remove excess water from your hair. The towel should be used lightly on your hair. This will protect your hair from split ends and breakage.

2. It is important to keep your hair clean. However, you should not shampoo it every day. If you use certain ingredients, such as shampoos that call for cold water, rinse your hair with warm water. Avoid using hot water on your hair as it can cause dryness and irritation.

3. Carefully choose your hair brushes and combs. Make sure to choose natural materials. You should not touch your scalp with the product. It will allow you to have fun while regulating blood flow. When untangling your tresses, you can use a wide toothed comb. It causes less friction and is gentle on your scalp.

4. You should air dry your hair and avoid styling it with hair dryers. Your hair can be permanently damaged by artificial heat. These can damage hair and make it weaker, more fragile, and more rough.

5. All hair tools should be kept clean and tidy. You should never give other people your combs, brushes, or other essentials for styling your hair.

6. A good hair massage should be done at least once every week. You can use either your favourite natural oils or commercially available hair masks. Massage your hair and leave it on for 30 minutes to overnight. This will help improve the blood circulation to your scalp and gives your hair extra shine.

7. Water is essential. This is a good habit to have for your entire body. This helps to keep your scalp and body hydrated. It's a natural way to moisturize your hair without any need for commercial products. This combination can be combined with eating healthy food such as fruits and vegetables to reap the benefits.

These are the do's and don'ts when it comes to hair care.

1. Don't comb your locks fast, even if it is urgent. Be patient and untangle your hair using a wide-toothed brush or your fingers. After that, you can gently brush the comb or brush through your hair.

2. You should not pull your hair tighter than necessary. This will cause hair to become brittle and can also damage your scalp. The hairstyles you choose should complement your style, so don't use tight braids.

3. You shouldn't always use your blow dryer on hair. It is better to let your hair air dry. It is best to keep the hair dry between the dryer's head and the scalp. Do not leave too much heat on the same area for too long. Use the lowest temperature setting possible and limit the heat for as long as you can.

4. Laureth Sulfates can cause hair loss and allergic reactions. It is safer and easier to use all-natural hair products.

It is important to follow the basic steps for hair care. This will ensure that your hair stays healthy and is not damaged. This can slow down the aging process.

## Chapter 11: Herbs And Mental Health For Mental Health Function

A variety of natural herbs can be used to keep your mind alert and healthy. These herbs are scientifically proven effective and can make you productive and healthy. You can make a huge difference by choosing from many of these suggested herbs.

Ginseng

This herb has been proven to increase memory and mental performance. Additionally, it can stimulate the immune system and lower blood cholesterol. Ginseng has been shown to be effective in anxiety treatment and improving resilience to stress and depression. Women and men who have taken ginseng herb have demonstrated greater resilience to stress and depression.

Ginseng root can be found in panaxosides as well as ginsenosides. These active ingredients are responsible for the healing properties. You can use this herb to fight fatigue, stress and cholesterol levels. It also helps prevent infections.

Being mentally healthy is an important factor in anti-aging. Ginseng can help reduce blood stream degeneration and improve mental performance.

Kudzu

Kudzu herb also known as Japanese Arrowroot, is highly recommended, especially if your goal is to reduce alcohol consumption and the death of brain cells. The herb regulates alcohol intake through brain communication, alerting it that an appropriate amount is required. This herb will prevent you from drinking excessive amounts of alcohol. In fact, binge-drinkers can actually reduce their alcohol intake by taking an extract of the kudzuvine for 7 days.

Active ingredients like puerarin in Kudzu also help to increase blood flow, especially in times of emergency.

Chamomile

This herb is very effective at reducing stress, nerve pain, and cramps. Chamomile can also be taken in the form of herbal teas or applied topically. It is recommended that you consume 9-15g daily. Chamomile oils contain a-bisabolol and farnesene. They have anti-inflammatory as well as antispasmodic properties.

The best way to get the herb is to make tea with it. It will reduce tension and help maintain brain health. For a relaxing effect, warm concoctions are best.

Holy Basil

Holy basil, also known by the name tulsi can reduce stress levels by inhibiting cortisol build-up. This herb can increase cerebral circulation and memory. It also helps with mental fog and cloudy thinking. Treatments for attention deficit disorder, attention-deficit hyperactivity disorder, and other forms of depression include holy basil. Holy basil leaf extract can be used in combination with silymarin. This active ingredient is made of several flavonoids.

Bacopa

Bacopa, which is indigenous to India, has been found to be highly effective in improving memory and learning. It contains active ingredients, including triterpene glycosides. This herb can improve your memory. This substance boosts the efficiency of nerve impulses transmission.

Bacopa's antioxidant properties offer brain protection.

The benefits of taking a bacopa oil herbal extract include improved cognitive function, focus, emotional well being and better memory.

Valerian

Valerian herb, a natural substance that occurs naturally, is an effective treatment for insomnia. It works better than conventional sleeping pills and doesn't have side effects. Valerian root contains isovaltrate. It is an active ingredient known for its medicinal benefits. Valerian root is a soothing and sedative herb that can help with insomnia and sleeplessness.

Valerian root is a good choice because it doesn't cause sleepiness and drowsiness during daylight hours. The root is also a muscle relaxant that can be used to reduce muscle spasms, cramps, and stiffness.

Herbs for Reproductive Health

Although many of us don't like to discuss our reproductive health, this is an important part our lives. Here are some effective herbs to improve your overall reproductive health.

Chaste Berry

Chaste Berry is small and peppery-tasting, and can be used by females to regulate hormonal levels. Premenstrual symptoms include breast pain, tenderness, mood swings, irritability and headaches.

The herb can also be used for other conditions such as premenstrual dysphonic disorder. This is a more severe form of premenstrual syndrome. Oral administration of this herb is effective for infertility treatment. It can be especially useful for infertile women because it can boost the progesterone hormone that regulates pregnancy. For 3-7 weeks, you can take the herbal extract to enhance the chance of having a baby.

Saw Palmetto

This herb is highly effective in maintaining good health for the prostate and relieving symptoms of an over-enlarged prostate. This problem is common in men over 50 years old. It can cause urination difficulties and swelling of the lower pelvis or rectal region. This herb can also be used as an aphrodisiac for impotence and as a sexual rejuvenator.

Saw Palmetto prevents dihydrotestosterone stimulating cell production in the prostate cells. Stimulating the prostate cells will be possible by blocking testosterone from binding. Saw palmetto prevents the proliferation of prostatic cells and thus reduces prostatic enlargement. It can also treat weak urinary systems in elderly women and men following menopause.

Daminana Leave

This herb is versatile and can be used to treat sex problems for men and women. It can also reduce the symptoms of menopause. The herb's medicinal properties ensure it is able to effectively boost libido as well as reproductive health. The herb's active constituents are effective in stimulating nerves, the reproductive system, blood circulation, and body metabolism.

The natural herb extract will boost libido and desire by increasing the oxygen supply to the genitalia. You can use the extract to treat erectile difficulties in men who have had repeated intercourses after an orgasm. This herb also has the ability to expand the blood vessels. This is necessary to ensure that men experience stable and consistent erections. This herb can enhance pleasure levels and increase a woman's ability to get orgasm.

Beth Root

When administered as an herbal tea, Beth root can be used to balance hormones. The ideal balance of hormones can help to ensure a normal cycle, easier pregnancy, and lower menopause effects. The root is known for its soothing and relaxing properties.

While Beth root action does not dry out the mucous membranes completely, it can control excess bleeding and reduce superfluous discharges. It is also a powerful remedy for hemorhages

Sea Buckthorn

The herb contains palmitoleic, which is why it's recommended for women who are suffering from vaginal dryness. This active ingredient is vital in keeping skin moist and the mucus membranes hydrated. Sea buckthorn oil is essential for providing essential nutrients to your body. The oil has many effects on the body's circulation, reproductive, endocrine and nerve systems. It also regulates and coordinates them.

A plant's ability to stop the growth and spread of microbes is another benefit that can be used for reproductive health. External and internal use of the oil has proved effective in treating vaginal, uterine, or cervical related problems. Sea Buckthorn is also very beneficial in maintaining smooth midlife and optimal performance for the uterus, while keeping the vagina moist.

## Chapter 12: Honey: The Lowdown

The National Honey Board states that one tablespoon of raw honey is entirely free of fat, cholesterol, sodium, and only 64 calories. Because of its widely-respected antibacterial, antifungal and medicinal properties, honey has been around since the Egyptian tombs. This golden fluid has a lot of health benefits that can help improve your health.

Beehives are not just a matter of humans. They have been there for many years. Beehives are a favorite target for many animals, such as bears and badgers. They provide a sweet treat that is delicious.

Honey was, in fact, the most common natural sweetener before sugar was made accessible to the general population.

How honey made

Before we begin, let us take a moment to look at the process of making honey.

It all begins with nectar

Honey starts with nectar from flowers. The nectar is collected and stored by bees in their honeycombs once it has been converted into simple sugars. Honey is produced when honeybees lift their wings, allowing the process of evaporate to occur.

Then comes the beekeepers

It is a good thing that bees can produce more honey per hive than they require. The honey we have left over is ours to use, and it's not something that we should feel guilty about. The beekeeper follows suit. They collect the honeycomb frames, and then remove the wax caps. The frames are then placed into an extractor which squeezes the honey out from the comb.

The final step

Finally, strain the honey to remove any waxy bits. Once the honey has been strained, it's time to bottle it and send it to the retailers. So that you can be certain that the honey you receive is pure, you might want to purchase a bottle.

## Chapter 13: All Natural Skin Remedies

These natural herbal remedies are versatile and can be used for many purposes. You'll find a solution for everything, even skin problems. These are great options for anyone who has suffered from skin allergies or bug bites that have reduced the skin's glow.

Bentonite Clay: Clay is great when you have itchy skin. It can also be used to treat acne breakouts. It can also be helpful in treating venomous bites/stings such as those from wasps, honeybees, and spiders. The clay pulls out the skin venom, and alleviates the pain. This helps the area heal quickly. How do I use it? You can use untreated clay also known as green or raw clay. This type of clay is the most powerful and heals the skin. You can mix it with a cup filtered water until you get a consistency that resembles peanut Butter. Then, simply apply the mixture on the affected area. After it dries, you can gently peel it away.

Also, you can make a clay packet. This would require you to spread the clay over a piece clean of porous material. You could use cotton, linen or flannel. After that, place the clay-covered cloth over the affected area. The clay should touch the skin. Allow it to dry for 4 hours or until it hardens.

Apple Cider Vinegar – This is not the first time you have heard about the incredible benefits of ACV. It's an effective antiseptic, and also contains antibacterial/antifungal agents. For example, sunburns and excessive dandruff. It's also used extensively for pets. Just add a cup to your pet's bath water. You can also use it on your skin by using a cotton towel and some of the vinegar to rub onto the area. The unfiltered and raw organic cider vinegar that is still strand-like sediments on the bottom of the bottles would be the best. This is because it will still contain all the beneficial enzymes for medicinal use.

Aloe Vera: Everyone knows aloe verde is great for skin. It can treat many skin irritations. It soothes the skin, reduces swelling, and moisturizes it. It is common to use it in natural lotions or creams. The best part? It is also quite common. Southern California residents have a 80% chance of finding one in their yard. How to use it Simply cut off the leaf and gently slice it along its length, starting at the top. Take the liquid from the leaf and rub it

onto your skin. Refrigerate any remaining gel. It
should last for one week.

## Chapter 14: Herbal Therapy

Herbal Therapy: A form of alternative medicine. Its history and uses. Herbal Therapy is a science that predates "conventional medicine" by thousands of year.

Herbal therapy may be called Herbal Medicine or Botanical Medicine or Herbology. It is all one thing, regardless of the name.

This alternative medicine uses plants in one form or another. It can also contain products from bees, minerals, and certain animals.

How herbal therapy works

Herbal medicine works in the same way as chemical medicines. While this implies that they can be equally effective, it can also mean they can cause damage. It is not all natural medicine that is healthy. You need to know the specific functions of each plant. The wrong plant can prove fatal. Although most people know the dangers associated with overdosing or using the wrong medication, many don't realize that natural products are just as dangerous.

Over the centuries, plants have come up with many methods of protecting themselves against predators (for instance animals and mushrooms) that can be very useful to us. There are approximately 12,000 known. However, this is only 10% of the total.

Animals seem able to "sense" what is good and what is bad for them. We humans don't have this sense. Also, animals are known to alter their eating patterns when they feel unwell. Unwell animals will eat plants with certain properties. Research shows this is because the plant's substance is important to them.

Every type of plant we eat around the globe has a beneficial property that will benefit us.

Herbal Therapy: A History

The use of plants to treat medical problems has been around as long the history of man.

After being found after having spent 5,300 years in an ice lake, "Otzi", the Iceman was examined. There were medicinal herbs that were discovered. These were likely used to treat a parasitic infection.

There are written records that Sumerians used laurel & thyme. Ancient Egyptians used mint, garlic, coriander & mint. These are just a handful of examples of early herbal use for healing and treating medical problems.

The Chinese herbal books of the 2700BC period contain a list listing 365 plants that were used for medicine. Each plant is also given uses.

Hippocrates (the founder of modern medicine) advocated the healing properties of herbs.

There were some problems in herbal medicine. One of the most well-known was towards the middle of the Middle Ages. Women who "cured with herbs" were persecuted and branded witches.

Plants were used to treat ailments. Trade opened up more exotic spices, herbs and herbs from other nations. The result was a greater variety of treatments.

The invention of printing led to the creation of many, many herbal book. This shows how popular this science was.

It was then that schools were established to teach herbs preparation and their use.

Chemical drugs were created in the 1500's to treat serious illnesses. It was estimated to have killed 30-60% in Europe.

Although mercury and arsenic were common chemical treatments at the time, they were not considered to be a cure-all. The dangers and toxins of these substances paled in comparison to the alternative of Syphilis dying.

Herbal Therapy Today

It is believed that 25% of modern medicine originates from traditional, herb-based medicine. About 80% use herbal medicine in some capacity.

Many spices and herbs used in seasoning food can have beneficial effects on your health.

It is estimated that 35,000 plants compounds have health value.

It is possible for a student to earn a degree in herbal medicine from a university. Governments take this seriously.

"Grow Your Own Drugs," a BBC series, proved to be very popular. Different health problems were addressed using plants from gardens and wild plants, as well as "recipes" that were made. Participants who could not find satisfactory treatments with conventional medication then tried the natural remedy and reported their results. Nearly every participant experienced some improvement. Some reported that they felt cured.

How herbs are used

You can use herbs in many different ways. In liquid form, such as tinctures. These are typically taken internally. Tisanes are made by heating the herbs with hot water. They can be consumed quickly and easily.

It is obvious that oils, creams or lotions are used for rubbing the skin. While steam inhalation is intended for sinus problems,

You can now find heat packs, herbal pillows, and a variety of herbal remedies. Many of them will not cause harm, and they are easy to use even if skeptical. Any aid to healing and feeling better should always be welcomed, no matter what source it comes from, as long as there is no risk. This includes herbs.

## Advantages

Growing your own can be free.

If medically administered correctly, the potential for adverse reactions are minimal.

Herbal medicine tends better to treat chronic conditions than chemical drugs

Plants can treat conditions that are not possible with conventional medicine.

## Side Effects

Research has shown that some plants are almost certain to cause side effects, especially if they are consumed in excessive amounts or for long periods.

* Comfrey

* Ginger

* Ginseng

* Goldenseal

* Liquorice root

* Senna

* St. John's wort

* Valerian

This doesn't mean that you should avoid certain plants.

The effects of herbs on other medications and drugs can be adverse. Talk to your doctor before using herbal treatments.

This article should not be interpreted as a substitute for expert medical advice. You should consult your physician before taking any steps to improve your health.

Some herbs and their uses

There are far too many herbs to mention them all here, especially since there are also other forms of alternative therapy. Here are some useful herbs along with some spices.

You can grow them, but the leaves, root, or any part of the plant are not edible. In most cases you can purchase pills containing this substance at a herbal shop.

Aloe Vera

Aloe Vera leaf extracts are a soothing balm that can be used on burns, wounds, or any other skin problem.

Burdock

Burdock is said to act as a diuretic, and help lower blood sugar.

Basil

Basil, taken orally, is anti-inflammatory and a liver tonic. It helps reduce motion sickness, cholesterol, high blood pressure, as well as low blood sugar. It also relieves oily skin, stress relief as well as tension, urinary problems, and constipation.

Basil is wonderful in salads, sandwiches, pesto, and when stuffing chicken.

## Bergamot

Bergamot can also be taken orally with Earl Grey Tea. It has antiseptic properties and helps to relieve oily skin, nausea as well as vomiting

## Chamomile

Chamomile can be described as a flower. It is often consumed as a cup of tea and used to relax and calm anxiety. It is used to help heal wounds, reduce inflammation, and decrease swelling.

## Cinnamon

Cinnamon, taken orally, is antibacterial and acts as a kidney tonic.

It is delicious in desserts as well as added to a cup if coffee.

## Cloves

Cloves can be used topically orally as an oil. Clove oil has antiseptic properties. It can relieve toothache and tension.

## Common Hollyhock

Common Hollyhock is believed by some to be a laxative. It also reduces inflammation.

## Echinacea

Echinacea, a plant that can be used to treat and prevent the flu and colds, is available in the form of a stalk, leaf, or root. Also useful for treating infections and healing wounds.

You should avoid using this herb in large quantities. Echinacea could cause allergic reactions in some people who are allergic or sensitive to plants from the daisy plant family.

## Eucalyptus

Warm water, add Eucalyptus and inhale. This is a good decongestant for Sinusitis.

## Feverfew

Feverfew is a plant. Feverfew is a leaf that can be used to treat and prevent migraines.

Some cases of side effects from mouth ulcers or digestive irritation have been noted. It is best to test the product first and then stop if you notice any unpleasant side effects.

## Garlic

Garlic cloves, and a root. Garlic is believed reduces cholesterol and blood pressure. It also has antimicrobial properties. A school of experts believes it can fight cancer.

Garlic is safe. However, garlic should not be consumed in large quantities before surgery.

Ginger

Ginger is a root. Ginger is an anti-inflammatory and antiseptic root that helps to ease nausea, motion sickness and stomach cramps.

Experts suggest that large quantities can lead to bloating and other adverse reactions. However, this is not yet confirmed by science so it is best to use sparingly.

Gingko

Ginkgo leaf has many uses, including for asthma, bronchitis. memory, fatigue, tinnitus, dementia, and other brain-related issues.

The seeds contain toxin. Use only the leaf.

Ginseng

Ginseng root is a great tonic for all ailments, however, it could cause high blood pressure.

Goldenseal

Goldenseal root has been used to treat skin and eye irritations and also for diarrhea.

However, it can cause serious side effects if taken in high amounts. Experts advise against this.

Jasmine

Jasmine, taken orally (such as Jasmine Tea), can help to reduce stress and tension.

Lavender

Lavender is antibacterial, antiseptic and disinfectant. It can also be used for stress relief, panic attacks relaxation, muscle spasms. arthritis, back pain, joint pain, mood enhancer.

Lavender is good in desserts.

Lemon Thyme

Lemon Thyme acts as a muscle relaxant, general tonic, and disinfectant.

Lemon Balm

Lemon Balm aids with overactive thyroid, panic attacks anxiety, relaxation, stress, sedatives tension, reducing tension headaches fevers and aiding in sleep.

Milk Thistle

Milk Thistle may be able to help your liver and lower cholesterol.

Mint

Mint helps digestion problems, peppermint gives extra energy, nausea, tension, arthritis, dandruff, joint pain

You can either buy drops or make your own mint tea. Or, you can add mint to any hot or cold water.

Mustard Seeds

Mustard Seeds may speed metabolism, decrease digestion, increase saliva production and help with migraines.

Nutmeg

Take Nutmeg to relieve nausea, rheumatism and muscle spasms

Parsley

Parsley can lower cholesterol

Rose

Rose flowers have anti-inflammatory properties.

Great tasting jams and desserts can be made with rose petals

Rosemary

Rosemary can either be taken orally or used as an oil for dandruff

This can help with aching joints as well as menopause hot flashes. It is also thought that it can aid Alzheimer's. It acts as a heart stimulant, gives extra energy, and helps to reduce or clear dandruff.

You can either buy it in concentrated form or make a Rosemary tea infusion by boiling fresh Rosemary. Even though Rosemary is a favorite, it doesn't taste very good. Buy drops and you can quickly take it all in one sitting.

Sage

Sage aids hot flushes, and generally during the menopause.

Saint John's Wort

Saint John's Wort's flowers and leaves can be used as an antidepressant.

Turmeric

Turmeric lowers cholesterol and fights fungal infection.

While these natural substances might be able to alleviate or help the mentioned conditions, it is important to seek professional help for more severe conditions.

Valerian

Valerian root is used as a natural remedy for insomnia and anxiety.

Valerian is used in America for flavoring root beer and other foods.

Violet

Violet aids sinus headaches and constipation

Witch Hazel

Witch Hazel creams and gels can be applied topically to soothe itching, burning, and some stings

You should always consult your healthcare provider before taking any of these herbs.

## Chapter 15: Herbs For Heart And Circulatory System

As the title indicates, these herbs can improve heart health and circulatory system.

Garlic

A garlic extract has been shown to reduce the risk of heart disease. Regular consumption of garlic can lower blood pressure and prevent cardiovascular disease. Garlic can be used to prevent cancer and kill bacteria.

Allicin, an antimicrobial substance in garlic, helps in reducing the risk of developing heart and circulatory disorders. Garlic can either be crushed, chewed raw garlic, or made into garlic juice in any form.

Cinnamon

According to scientific research, cinnamon can help lower blood sugar and keep cholesterol levels low. High blood pressure can be caused by high cholesterol levels.

Cinnamon has anti-clotting qualities that limit unwanted clumping. The heart may pump thicker blood under higher pressure if it is clumped. Cinnamon works better than aspirin. This drug produces a similar effect, but has some limitations. You can use cinnamon to spice up your food and reap the benefits.

Hawthorn

This flowering herb's flowers are used to treat heart issues such as lower blood pressure, slower heart beat, and unblocking of coronary arteries. This is because of a compound called vitexin-2" or rhamnoside. The treatment of heart problems can be improved by taking hawthorn herbs for at least 6 months. You can also use it to treat the early stages of heart disease without having to take any medication.

Heart failure refers to a lack of blood supply to the heart. Heart failure can lead to fatigue, fluid retention and shortness of breath. Hawthorn can help with the problem.

Dandelion

The herb also grows as an herb and is highly effective in controlling blood sugar. Researchers include active ingredients in drugs such as sesquiterpene lintones from the Dandelion root.

Dandelion root can be taken to lower blood volume. This will effectively lower blood pressure and reduce water retention. Flavonoids as well as polyphenols, which are antioxidants that can promote heart health, are some of the benefits this herb offers. This herb can help with problems such as heartburn, kidney disease, or other digestive issues.

Cayenne pepper

Cayenne pepper has a high level of cardiovascular health benefits. The active ingredient capsicum stimulates the work of this herb. Cayenne can help prevent heart attacks, alleviate plagues, improve blood circulation and nourish the body with nutrients.

Cayenne is also known to lower blood pressure, improve blood vessel flexibility and reduce bleeding. Cayenne pepper Powder can be made with hot chili peppers. It's rich in more 26 active nutrients like selenium.

Herbs for the Urinary and Digestive System

For optimal physical health, you should take the following herbs:

## Ginger

It is recommended to ginger if you suffer stomach upsets. This slows down production of serotonin. This substance is responsible for nausea and motion sickness, as well as other issues during pregnancy. Ginger tea is rich in phenolic compounds like gingerol or shagaol. It also contains organic oils, which makes it extremely effective in the digestion system.

Ginger tea is excellent for stomach gas, flatulence and treating heartburn. The active ingredients of ginger may help to lower the acid reflux rate by inhibiting acid.

## Uva Ursi

Uva Ursi herbs can be very beneficial for people suffering from urinary tract infection, such as bladder disease and kidney disease. Uva Ursi herb is rich in enzymes that secrete the glucoside-arbutin, a very absorbable compound that your kidneys need for fighting bacterial infections. Glucosade arcbutin is secreted by the body during the production of urine. This helps to kill and treat microorganisms.

Uva Ursi may also be used to treat conditions such as cystgisis or urethritis. You can get rid of bladder stones and uric Acid accumulation. A recommended dosage of the herb is 400 to 840 mgs of glucoseside arbutin, for approximately two weeks.

Licorice

This herb is popular for its sweet taste. However, it also has amazing healing properties that are helpful in many digestive issues. Licorice has the ability to soothe and relax your gastrointestinal tissues. This is especially useful if you suffer from acid reflux or ulcer pain.

Glycyrrhizin in licorice leaves contains healing properties. Making herbal tea with licorice involves grinding the roots and adding them to your preferred beverage, such as tea or coffee.

Celery seed

Celery seeds are a good choice for people who experience persistent problems when they urinate. They have excellent diuretic properties. Celery seeds have a number active ingredients including coumarins. flavonoids. and volatile oils. They are also healing agents.

They are also diuretic and can be used to treat excess urination. Toxins such accumulated uric acids are removed along with problems like kidney stones and water retention.

Milk Thistle

This herb is very effective in stimulating the regeneration of your liver tissue. It also maintains the optimal functions of your liver. The active ingredient that protects the liver is silymarin which is found in milk thistle. The silymarin compound, a group of flavonoids, repairs liver cells from damage by alcohol or other toxic substances.

Flavernoids help to protect the liver's new cells from toxic substances and also reduce inflammation. You can make a liquid extract, or a tincture from milk thistle to prepare a nutritious drink. To make atincture, grind the seeds of this herb and mix it with alcohol or another solvent. If you have a liver condition that is related to alcohol, avoid making an alcohol tincture.

## Chapter 16: Herbals For Weight Loss

With new products coming on the market daily, weight loss is a multi-billion dollar business. These products don't always deliver and they can actually be a waste of money. As if all that weren't bad enough many of these so-called "weight loss pills" can contain potentially dangerous ingredients that cause more harm then good. There are safer, more natural alternatives. This is where herbs come into play.

Weight loss can be promoted by several inexpensive and readily accessible herbs. However, the following herbs aren't going to make you lose weight overnight. When combined with exercise and a healthy diet, the herbs can help you lose weight.

Cinnamon

One of the most popular herbs for weight loss is cinnamon according to herbalists. It helps you feel fuller for longer times, slows down fat metabolization, reduces hunger pangs, stabilizes blood sugar, and keeps you satisfied.

Ginger

Ginger is a natural cleanser and can help to get rid of any food stuck in your system. This will prevent you from storing fat and reduce your weight gain.

## Turmeric

Turmeric is a yellowish orange-colored spice with weight loss properties. Turmeric has been shown to decrease fat tissue formation. This in turn helps prevent weight gain.

## Cardamom

Cardamom has been shown in studies to increase metabolism and burn fat.

## Dandelion

Despite being labeled a weed, dandelion actually flowers and can cleanse the body. They also have high nutritional content, which can make you feel fuller over a longer time.

## Mustard

This herb is known to boost metabolism.

## Guarana

Guarana's high caffeine content gives it its weight-loss effect. It is also stimulant and diuretic.

It is important to remember that guarana, a stimulant herb, should not be taken if you are already taking other stimulant herbs and medications. It could increase your blood pressure.

Herbal Teas for Weight Loss

Because teas have less side effects and are quicker than unhealthy chemical slimming pill alternatives, they are very popular. You should drink those teas as part of a balanced diet, and exercise regularly.

Inadequate quantities can lead to people believing that quality is more important than quantity. Common complaints when drinking excessive weight loss teas include nausea, diarrhea, and headaches.

Moderation is important. Although some teas may be helpful in weight loss, it should not be taken as the sole solution. It is better to stick with a weight loss plan. The combination of different weapons will be beneficial. Natural weight loss herbal teas can also help to shed unwanted pounds.

Get slimmer by following my top tips.

Green Tea

This is a common one. I'm sure you've heard it before. Green tea is a popular choice for natural weight loss due to its strong thermogenesis properties. Its Catechin (EGCG), which is a powerful preventative against cancer, is also touted as a strong fat burner. It increases internal temperature, which in turn enhances metabolism.

You can stimulate your metabolism by simply drinking green tea each day. It also provides powerful antioxidants.

Red tea as well as green tea can be used to burn fat. It is possible to substitute at least one cup per day of coffee with green tea. This will help you feel healthier and more energetic over the long term. Green tea is a good source of some levels, but not as stimulating as coffee.

While coffee may give you an immediate energy boost, coffee will soon cause you to become dependent on it. Green tea offers a subtler, longer-lasting, mental and physical stimulation. It is also not affected by an abrupt decrease in energy.

## Peppermint Tea

This tea is great for relieving strong cravings. It works as an appetite suppressant. This helps to eliminate unwanted cravings that can lead to poor diet. This can also be very helpful if you have a poor digestion. Mint tea is a wonderful addition to green tea. You will get an antioxidant-rich, naturally revitalizing drink that was traditionally known as the

Moroccan tea. Although it is tempting to make your green or mint tees sweeter than the Moroccans, you should be careful. You are trying to lose weight. If you add mint herbs to your green tea or a mint tea bag, you can make it sweeter and more appealing. It will also help you to resist the temptation to consume sugar.

## Oolong Tea

Oolong mushrooms are a type used to treat a variety of medical conditions including heart disease, tooth decay, and osteoporosis. It is an effective weight loss tea that reduces cholesterol levels, stimulates metabolism, increases fat consumption, and also makes it easier for muscles to use fats more efficiently. Oolong tea is rich in caffeine, which stimulates central nervous system. You should avoid oolong or reduce the amount you drink if your body is sensitive to caffeine.

Star Anise Tea - The Chinese Star Anise Species

It isn't my favourite tea but it is very effective in weight loss efforts. It aids in digestion, making it easier to expend fats and water. The tea stimulates the slow lymphatic system, which can be a problem if you have trouble eliminating water retention. It stimulates the elimination and recovery of toxins.

You should research the brand before you buy the Chinese Star Anise. This is because the Japanese is toxic to your health and shouldn't be eaten.

Star anise has been used by many phytotherapists for the treatment of flu, rheumatism and inflammation. It's also used extensively in Vietnamese and Chinese cuisines. The thing I find most fascinating about all natural remedies, is their versatility and the endless amount of information available. Also, I have a lot of respect for phytotherapists or herbalists. This is a lifetime-long process.

Rose Tea

It does more than simply relax the mind with the wonderful aroma. It also relaxes and prepares the muscles for tomorrow's fight. It's rich in vitamins-A and B3, C, D., E. This tea is great for weight loss.

It is also known to cleanse the liver and gall bladder, which promotes bile circulation. Rose tea is widely used as an Ayurvedic remedy. It is known to be an excellent antioxidant. Rose tea can be a good option for anyone who experiences fluid retention and general tiredness.

It is a wonderful choice for anyone suffering from stress or insomnia due to its calming effects. Personally, I find its aroma and flavor to be extremely relaxing. This multifunctional remedy is also great for its therapeutic properties.

To ensure you are able to make different types of teas, experiment with them. Tea can also be drunk cold. This allows you to enjoy a delicious, healthy energy drink.

For smoothies, you can also use teas like green tea, mint tea or rose water. If you cool down green tea, mint or rose tea, it can make a great base for smoothies.

Have you ever tried green-tea + strawberries + cherry + pineapple + a banana smoothie? It is a powerful weight loss stimulant, as well as being great for cellulite prevention and slowing down the flow of blood.

Juices for Weight Loss

Juicing vegetables, fruits, and herbs is a way to lose weight and keep a desirable body. It revolves around the principles detoxification as well as meal replacement.

Weight loss juices have the best ingredients for weight maintenance. These juices not only have fat burning and appetite suppressing capabilities, but are also rich with nutrients that are essential in maintaining your health while the physical changes take place. Why would you want to supplement your weight loss with juices when you already have all the supplements and teas you need?

First, juices as well as smoothies are meal replacements. These meals can help you keep something in your belly while also consuming less unhealthy processed food. Eat wisely, not just eat. Eating or drinking liquid meals is the best way to do this. You can drastically reduce your risk of having food cravings. Vegetable juices will give you energy, as well as prevent many serious diseases.

The second is that juices are a great detoxifier to get rid of all the toxins in your body. Particularly green smoothies will make you feel younger and help you look younger. What does detoxification mean for weight loss?

If the liver, along with other digestive organs, is full of toxins, then fat cannot burn calories and convert them into energy. For optimal metabolism to be restored, it is necessary to restore the liver's optimal function.

Finally, you can extract the natural weight-loss properties of fruits and herbs. Juicing is the best method to do that.

There are so many options for smoothies and juices.

For those who are looking to lose weight or rejuvenate their bodies, here are some tips for making smoothies and juices.

-Use only organic fruits & vegetables. You want to revitalize your body, so you don't need any artificial food preservatives.

Avoid procrastination. Although juicing and smoothie making may seem slow at first, you will see long-term results. You will avoid many conditions such as low energy, and possibly even need to visit the doctor. Make sure you remember to take time to look after your health each time you make a juice. There is no reason to lose one single day of life. You will also save money. Juicing is the best beauty treatment you can get, and it's all natural.

You and your partner will spend a lot together, so be sure to pick up a juicer as well as a blender. A blender that works well is just as important as a reliable car. It is worth looking into a juicer or blender with a long life span that can withstand the weight of your juice, as well as one that is easy to clean. I use Omega.

- You can buy juicers if your dislike making them. How often have you ordered a drink or a mug of coffee from a bar? There are many places offering fresh juices and smoothies.

What should you juice/blend

An experienced "juicing expert" would state that you can juice anything.

You can achieve balance, health, weight loss and health by eating high-alkalizing, low-sugar, high-mineral fruits and veggies.

Juicing Ingredients:

1. Alkaline veggies: cucumber, carrot, tomato, green spinach, broccoli, and onion. Juicing should focus on vegetables and leafy greens, so that you can concentrate your juice.

2. These alkaline fruit juices include grapefruit, lemons, limes, tomatoes, and pomegranates. Why? They are very low in sugar and extremely high in minerals. This makes them highly alkalizing, even though the taste is acidic.

If the alkaline Diet is new to you (it may sound complicated or even faddish at first), download your free eBooks. They include simple, printable charts.

Blending/Smoothie Ingredients:

Other fruits (here I mean fruits with low sugar content, such as bananas or kiwis) are acceptable. However, you shouldn't juice them. Instead blend them. Make tasty and colorful smoothies with them. If you want to lose weight, focus 80% on juicing vegetables, or using them for smoothies, and 20% on fruits that are low in sugar.

They could be used as a natural, healthy treat like kiwis, bananas or pineapples.

Additional suggestions:

You can also make your smoothies with coconut water, coconut water, ricemilk, oat milk and almond milk (super-alkaline!).

Alfalfa powder, soya levithin granules, and barleygrass can be useful additions to juices and smoothies.

## Chapter 17: Taheebo's Dangers

Although Taheebo tea is commonly associated with the idea it does not cause any side-effects and can be consumed in excess, this could lead to some serious medical problems. Supplement production differs from drug production in that producers of supplements don't need to prove effectiveness or safety to the Food and Drug Administration. It is possible to question the safety or effects of certain ingredients contained in a container.

Supplements of this type have not been tested against medications, so their interactions with medicines, foods, and other supplements are unclear. Although reports may indicate that side effects can occur, studies on interactions and effects of these supplements are rare. Taheebo usage can lead to side-effects that could, in certain cases, be very serious.

Anemia is one such side-effect. Anemia is when there is a decrease in red cell count in the body. This causes your body to not get enough oxygen which in turn can cause other serious problems. Apart from these, taheebo causes blood thinning and increases the possibility of bleeding and other abnormalities. Taheebo tea should not be consumed by anyone with an anticoagulant condition. These medications can include heparin and warfarin as well as nonsteroidal anti-inflammatory drug (such as ibuprofen. Warfarin has been shown to cause bleeding complications in combination with taheebo. Other drugs that can cause similar reactions include enoxaparin potassium and dalteparin. Aspirin has anticoagulant benefits by inhibiting platelet aggregation. Patients suffering from blood clots and those with a family history of bleeding should consult a doctor before using taheebo. It prevents blood from clotting, which could cause serious damage to tumors.

Some chemicals in taheebo, like hydroquinone are toxic. High doses of Taheebo Tea may damage the kidneys and liver. Research on rats has shown that mothers who were given Taheebo tea during pregnancy either lost their babies or gave rise to deformed babies. It is best to avoid taheebo while pregnant or breastfeeding. It is not known whether the same reaction will occur in humans.

Taheebo, like other popular herbal remedies, can cause allergic reactions. PDRhealth.com lists several signs, such as difficulty breathing, chest discomfort, tightness, pain in the chest or throat, rash or hives, or itchy, swollen skin. Additionally, allergic reactions such as those mentioned above are signs of a medical emergency that require immediate medical attention.

American Cancer Society has reaffirmed their opposition to taheebo-tea as "not available evidence from well designed, controlled studies supports this substance as an efficacious treatment for human cancer". As a treatment for any cancer, it is best to avoid or delay standard medical care and to rely solely on taheebo.

# Chapter 18: Herbal Remedies

Simple recipes, basic kitchen tools, as well as a well-stocked herb pharmacy, can make it easy to treat even the most serious ailments. This site has a lot of useful remedies.

Abscess

Abscess means an inflamed, infected area that is painfully hot. The more severe an abscess becomes, the more it will hurt. You should seek medical attention immediately if you aren't able to heal the abscess.

Agrimony-Chamomile Oil

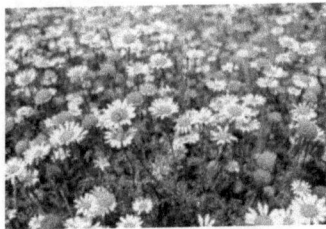

Makes approximately 2/3 cup.

Aloe Vera gel is combined with chamomile and Agrimony to reduce inflammation and soothe redness. The gel can be stored in the refrigerator. It can be kept fresh up to two weeks by being stored in an airtight container.

Ingredients:

* 1/2 to ¾ cup water

* 2 teaspoons dried Agrmony

* 1/4 cup aloe vera gel.

* 1 to 2 teaspoons dry chamomile

Instructions:

1. Combine the chamomile, agrimony, and water in a saucepan. Bring the mixture up to a boil, then reduce heat to medium. Boil the mixture on high heat until it reduces half. After that, remove from heat and let cool completely.

2. Use a piece of cheesecloth to dampen the funnel. Put the mixture into a glass bowl through the funnel. Use the funnel to squeeze out any liquid remaining from the herbs. Now, squeeze the cheesecloth again and squeeze the excess liquid out.

3. Mix the aloe gel with the liquid. Use a whisk for blending. Transfer the gel to sterilized glass jars. Seal the jar with a lid and place in the refrigerator.

4. Two times daily, use a cotton cosmetic cloth to apply a thin layer to affected areas.

Precautions

Allergies

Allergies refer to abnormal immune responses to common substances such as dust, pollen, or cat dander. Food, drinks, and even the environment can all contain allergens. It's not always possible to avoid them. While conventional treatments can suppress your body's immune response to allergens that are harmful, herbal remedies are much gentler.

# Echinacea & Goldenseal Tincture

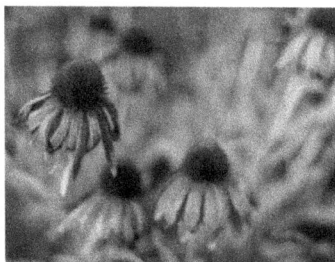

About 2 cups.

Echinacea or goldenseal are strong antibacterial agents that can boost your natural immune system. To ensure you always have it available, make the tincture in advance. It will last up to 7 year if stored in a dark and cool place. It is safe to use whenever you have an infectious condition.

Ingredients:

* 2 cups unflavored 80 proof vodka

* 4 ounces of dried echinacea roots, finely chopped

\* 2 to 3 ounces of dried goldenseal Root, finely chopped

Instructions:

1. In a pint jar sterilized, combine the goldenseal with the echinacea. Combine the vodka with the goldenseal and echinacea.

2. Close the lid and shake the jar. For 6-8 weeks, store it in a dark cabinet. Add vodka to the jar until it reaches the top.

3. Use cheesecloth to dampen a funnel. You can then pour the tincture through the funnel and into another pint-sized jar. Take the liquid from the roots and squeeze it out. Then, use the cheesecloth to remove any liquid. You can discard the roots and transfer the tincture into dark-colored glass containers.

4. You can treat an abscess by taking 10 drops orally, two to three times per day for 7-10 days.

Precautions Be aware that goldenseal can lower blood sugar and should be avoided if your diabetes is present.

Acne

Achy pimples result from red, swollen glands. While this is a common condition that affects teenagers, adults can get it. It doesn't matter if the acne affects just your face, or whether it has spread to your chest or back, herbal remedies can help you look and live better.

# Calendula Toner

This makes approximately 1/2 cup.

Calming calendula is used to reduce swelling. This simple toner also contains witch hazel which fights bacteria, while soothing your skin. This toner lasts at least one year when kept in a dark, cool area.

Ingredients:

* 1 to 2 tablespoons calendula olive oil

* ½ to 1/3 cup witch hazel

Instructions:

1. Mix all ingredients together in a dark glass bottle and shake the bottle gently.

2. Apply five to six drops to your freshly cleaned face. As needed, add more or less.

3. Repeat the procedure twice daily while your acne remains. You can store the bottle in a refrigerator if it gives you a cooling sensation.

# Feverfew Peppermint Tincture

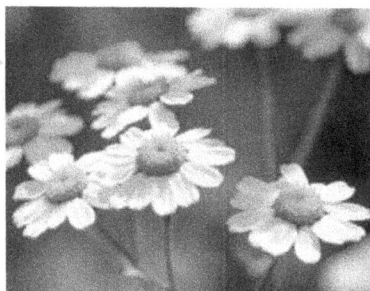

About 2 cups.

When you suffer from an allergy attack, peppermint or feverfew help open your airways. Peppermint is a good alternative to feverfew. The tincture will last up to 7 year if stored in a cool, dark area.

Ingredients:

* 5 to 6 ounces dried peppermint

* 1 to 2 ounces dried feverfew

* 2 to 2 ½ cups unflavored 80proof vodka

Instructions:

1. Combine the peppermint powder and the feverfew in an sterilized pint-jar. Fill the jar with vodka.

2. Close the lid and shake the jar. For 6-8 weeks, store it in a cool dark cabinet.

3. Use cheesecloth to dampen a funnel. Place the tincture in a funnel and transfer it into another pint-jar. You can then squeeze the liquid out of the herbs. You can discard the herbs, and you can transfer the tincture into dark-colored glass bottles.

4. You can take 5 drops orally if you are experiencing allergy symptoms. Mix the liquid with water or juice if the taste is too strong.

Take precautions: If you have an allergy to ragweed, feverfew should not be used. Feverfew should be avoided during pregnancy.

# Fresh Yarrow Poultice

Makes 1 poultice.

Yarrow contains anti-inflammatory compounds and antibacterial substances. It helps to reduce inflammation, swelling, and speed up healing.

Ingredients:

* 1 cup finely chopped fresh yellow arrow leaves

Instructions:

1. After applying the chopped leaves to your abscess, cover it with a moist cloth. Keep the poultice on for at least 10 to 15 min.

2. Repeat the procedure two to three more times per day until you feel your abscess is gone.

Use during pregnancy with caution People allergic to Asteraceae can have skin reactions from yarrow.

# Ginkgo and Thyme Tea

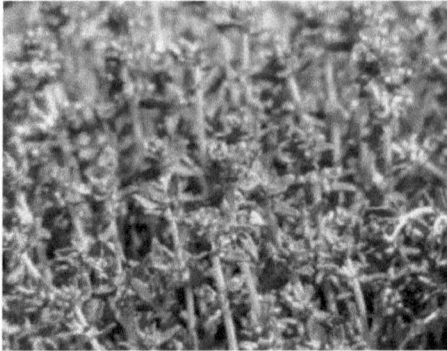

Makes 1 cup

Ginkgo biloba (thyme) and ginkgo biloba open your airways to allow you to breathe more easily. If you don't like the flavor of this tea you can add a teaspoon honey or dried mint to enhance its taste.

Ingredients:

* 1 cup boiling Water

* 1 to 1 ½ teaspoon dried Gingo biloba

* 1 to 2 teaspoon dried mint.

Instructions:

1. Place the boiling water in large mug. Add the dried herbs to the mug. Let the tea steep for 10 mins.

2. After relaxing, take a sip of the hot tea and inhale the steam. Repeat it four times a day.

Safety precautions: If you have monoamine oxide inhibitor (MAOI), prescriptions for depression, do not consume this tea. The effects of blood thinners are increased by Ginkgo biloba, so consult your doctor before taking this tea.

Foot of an Athlete

This fungus causes a scratchy, sometimes aching, infection that can be painful and it thrives in damp, warm, dark environments. Make sure to get rid of it before it spreads to your toenails. This can lead to discoloration and disfigurement which is very difficult for you to fix.

# Fresh Garlic Poultice

Takes only 1 treatment

Garlic is a powerful antifungal that can be used to eliminate athlete's heel. Raw honey can help bind the garlic and provide additional antifungal activity. Although it is possible for you to make a double, triple or even triple batch of this remedy over the course 2 to 3 day period, you might be able to achieve quicker healing by making a fresh batch each time.

Ingredients:

* 1 to 1 ½ garlic clove, pressed

1 teaspoon raw honey

Instructions:

1. Combine the honey with the garlic in a small container. Apply the blend to the skin using a cotton cosmetic pads.

2. Slip on a pair if clean socks and then let your feet relax for between 15 minutes and an hour. Afterward, dry your feet. Continue the treatment for at least two more times per day. Apply

Goldenseal Ointment to your feet (HERE). Continue for 3 days after symptoms disappear.

Garlic could cause a skin reaction in sensitive people.

## Ointment with Goldenseal

This makes about 1 to 2 cup.

Goldenseal can be used to prevent athlete's heel. You can use this ointment by itself or with the Fresh Garlic Poultice. The ointment can be kept fresh up to a year if it is kept in a dark and cool place.

Ingredients:

* 1-ounce beeswax

* 1 to 1 ½ cup light olive oil

* 2 to 3 ounces dried goldenseal root, chopped

Instructions:

1. Combine the olive oils and goldenseal in slow cooker Set the lowest heat setting. Cover the slow cooker. Allow the roots to steep in oil for 3 to 5 hours. Let the oil cool down before you turn off the heat.

2. Bring the water to a boil in the bottom of a double-boiler. Reduce the heat down to low.

3. Put a piece if cheesecloth over half the boiler. The infused oil should be poured into the

cheesecloth. Twist the cheesecloth until it is completely dry. Toss the cheesecloth with the herbs that have dried.

4. The infused oil can be added to the beeswax. Heat gently at low heat. After the beeswax melted completely in the pan, turn off the heat. Do not hesitate to pour the mixture into clean, dry glass jars or tins. Allow it to cool completely before covering.

5. You can apply 1/4 teaspoon to each of the affected areas using a cotton makeup pad. You can apply a little more or less depending on the area. To prevent slipping, wear a pair clean socks on top of the ointment.

Precautions You have high blood Pressure?

# Garlic-Ginkgo Syrup

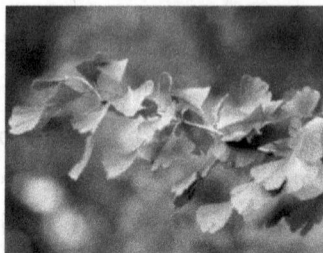

About 2 cups.

Ginkgo biloba has more than a dozen antihistamine constituents. Garlic can boost your immune system. It is worth using local honey, as it can help you build resistance to allergens from your area. Refrigerated syrup will keep for at least 6 months.

Ingredients:

* 2 to 2 ½ ounces ginkgo Biloba, crushed or chopped

* 2 to 3 ounces fresh, frozen or dried garlic chopped

* 1 to 2 cups water

* 1 cup of local honey

Instructions:

1. Combine the water, garlic, and ginkgo biloba in an saucepan. Bring the liquid up to a simmer, reduce heat to low, cover with a lid, then reduce liquid by half.

2. Take the contents of a saucepan and pour it into a glass measuring bowl. Then, place a portion of the mixture on a dampened cloth.

3. Heat the honey in a saucepan. Stir continuously and then reduce heat to low.

4. Put the syrup in a sterilized jar/bottle and keep it in your refrigerator.

5. You can take one teaspoon orally three times daily until your allergies disappear.

Precautions: Do NOT use if your monoamine oxidase inhibit (MAOI), is being used to treat depression. Ginkgo Biloba is a blood thinner that improves the outcome. Please consult your doctor before you use it. Children under the age of 12 should not take more than 1 teaspoon per day.

## Asthma

This chronic condition causes inflammation in the lungs and constrictions of the bronchial tubes. Asthma attacks may be frightening. People can also experience panic attacks when their breathing becomes difficult.

## Chapter 19: Medicinal Herb Garden

It's a good idea to make your own herbal remedies. You can also save money by growing your herbs and spices. It doesn't matter if you are a beginner or an experienced gardener. Many herbs are very hardy and can be grown in either a container, a greenhouse or a flowerbed.

While most plants can be found in supermarkets or garden centres, you can purchase seeds for very little money if the plant is something that interests you. Or, save the seeds you use for your daily cooking and make your own herb garden.

Personal choice will determine how many herbs and how much space is needed. However, herbs thrive in all kinds of environments so you can use planters and window boxes if you do not have enough garden space.

A benefit of growing medicinal herbs is their versatility. They can also be used to make delicious dishes.

The best herbs are ready to pick when they are at the peak of their potential. This can give your home a rustic look. Do not waste the herbs. Use what you can and hang the rest up to dry. This will not only ensure you have enough medicinal ingredients on hand for when you need them, but it will also look fantastic and add wonderful scents to the home.

Many herbs grow well indoors and outside, so you can scatter some potted herbs all around your house and bring some nature into your home.

Getting Started

If you are new to growing herbs, it is a good idea to start small with 5-10 plants and then build up your herb gardens. If your plants don't thrive, it is important to not get discouraged.

The key to understanding your plants is to learn their likes and dislikes, what they are used to, and whether they prefer the sun or the shade.

Experiment and practice. Every year you fail a plant, you'll learn something new and will be ready to plant the next one. The only thing that can cause a plant to die is not what you have done. It could be anything from the environment, the temperature and humidity, or even the soil you use. It is a living creature and as such, they are subject to environmental changes.

Remember that soil is essential for plants to thrive. So invest in quality compost. And most importantly, have patience. You can expect plants to start appearing after 3 weeks if you plant them from seed. The process of growing plants from seed takes time. Learn as much as you can about your plants before you begin to plant them.

Plants

Below is a listing of plants that you can consider including in your herb gardens. Pick the herbs you wish to begin with, from either the listed list or your own selection.

These herbs are relatively easy to grow, and they can provide a wonderful all-round medicinal garden.

* Basil

* Calendula

* Cayenne Pepper

* Chamomile

Chickweed

* Coriander

* Dill

* Echinacea

* Feverfew

* Garlic

* Ginger

* Lavender

* Lemon Balm

* Marjoram

* Mint

* Rosemary

* Sage

* Thyme

* Valerian

All plants, with the exception of Yarrow & Valerian, are able to grow well in either flowerbeds or containers, save for Valerian & Yarrow.

Design

If you have the space to do so, it is worth thinking about how you can design your medicinal herb gardens in a way that adds interest and allows you to keep the plants together.

The ladder and wagon wheel are two classic, stylish designs. You can place an old ladder or wagon wheel on your planting area. Each rung can be used to plant a different type of herb. The plants are separated, making it easier for you to identify and de-weed the herb beds.

## Chapter 20: Essential Oils

Essential oils are a traditional remedy that has been used to treat a variety ailments in the body since ancient times. Essential oils can not only make your home smell wonderful, but many others have more useful uses than that. They have the ability to heal both physically and emotionally. You can use them in the form of a diffuser or by directly applying them to your skin. Essential oils aren't oils at all, but highly concentrated plant components. The making of essential oils requires a lot more plants than usual, which can make them quite costly. This chapter will cover the top essential oils used, their uses, as well as a few recipe ideas to make your own.

Benefits of essential oil

* Balance hormones

* Aid to combat infection

* Increase overall immunity; speed up the recovery from illness

* Provide assistance to people in avoiding outdoor pests

Most Popular Essential Oils

Tea Tree

This oil can be applied topically. It's great for healing blemishes. You can use a cotton pad or a cottonball to apply the oil to your skin. It is likely to be in the list of skin care products already on your shelves.

Lavender

It can be used as a versatile oil and has calming effects to relax. It has the ability to heal minor cuts and irritations quickly. The aroma of lavender reduces stress hormones. When you next take a soak, add a few drops to the bathing water. You can even apply it to your skin or on your pillow before you go to sleep.

Calendula

Called also a "marigold," the bright orange colour of calendula makes it ideal for sensitive skin. It is known to reduce acne scars. It can also be used to soothe skin irritations related to psoriasis.

## Chamomile

Chamomile is often consumed in the form tea. This herb promotes relaxation.

## Peppermint

This oil can stimulate the mind and increase alertness mental. Studies have shown that peppermint inhalation can improve mental accuracy up to 28%.

## Frankincense

Another oil that can be used for relaxation is this one. It has been used to improve immunity, decrease inflammation and fight depression for thousands of year.

## Oregano

Although oregano can have a strong taste it is very effective in fighting off colds and other common ailments.

## Lemon

The great thing about lemon oil is its ability to detoxify the body. It is also great for fighting acne's peskiness. It can improve mental alertness as well as increase overall energy. This oil is ideal for those who feel tired and sluggish.

Grapefruit

Grapefruit oil works in the same way as lemon oil to reduce fatigue. It is also used in many home cleansers.

Eucalyptus

This is an essential oil that you can keep handy during the high allergy season. It can also help to combat congestion. It is also known to soothe sore muscles, and help build up your immune system.

Essential Oil Roller Recipes

Select a combination from the list below and combine them in a 10ml bottle. Simply shake the mixture!

* Tummy Tame: 8 droplets ginger, 10 droplets peppermint, 10 droplet lavender

* Mood Lifter: 5 droplet ylang ylang, 10 droplets bergamot, 10 droplets lavender

* Allergy Relief - 10 drops peppermint or lemon, 10 droplets lavender, 10 droplets lemon.

* Happiness blend: 5 drops lemon, 10 juniper berry drops, 10 juniper wild orange drops

* Muscle Rub: 5 droplets of clove, 5 droplets of black pepper and 10 droplets Wintergreen. 10 droplets Peppermint.

* Bruise Blend: 5 droplets fennel; 10 droplets helichrysum; 10 droplets lavender

* Stretch mark Stick: 5 droplets of Frankincense, 10 droplets Myrrh, and 15 droplets Lavender

* Blissful blend: 5 droplet lime, 5 droplets orange, 5 droplets red grapefruit, and 10 droplets of bergamot

* Cough Relief - 5 drops lemon, 10 droplets Frankincense, 15 drops Eucalyptus

* Headache Relief - 4 droplets frankincense; 10 droplets peppermint; 12 droplets lavender

* Blemish Stick: 5 droplets lavender, 10 droplets lemon, 10 droplets melaleuca, Jajoba carrier oil

* Focus Blend - 15 droplets wild orange and 15 droplets peppermint

* Natural Lip Gloss: 5 droplets lemon, 15 droplets lavender

* Fever Stick: 5 droplets frankincense, 10 droplets peppermint, 10 droplets lemon

* Cellulite Rub: 5 droplet lemon, 10 droplets rosemary, 15 droplets grapefruit

* Fatigue Fighter - 6 droplets grapefruit; 10 droplets rosemary; 14 droplets Eucalyptus

# * Razor Relief - 5 droplets Helichrysum, 5 drops Melaleuca and about 4 to 5 droplets Myrrh, 5 Droplets Frankincense, 5 Droplets Lavender.

* Tranquil Blend 5 droplets Bergamot, 5 droplets Yulang Ylang, 5 ylang ylang drops, 5 cypress droplets, 5 cypress droplets, 5 gallons sandalwood

* Sleepy Time Roller: 10 droplets chamomile, 10 droplets lavender, 10 droplets geranium

* Protective Blend: 5 droplets cinnamon, 5 droplets rosemary, 5 droplets eucalyptus, 5 droplets clove, 5 droplets lemon

* Stop Itching! 10 droplets peppermint, and 15 droplets lavender

* Healing Blend: 10 droplets lavender, 10 droplets melaleuca, 10 droplets frankincense

* Weight Loss Mix: 5 drops peppermint; 5 droplets ginger; 5 droplets cinnamon; 10 droplets lemon; 10 droplets grapefruit

* Memory Booster - 2 drops cinnamon, 5 droplets rosemary and 8 droplets lime, 10 droplets lavender

* Mental clarity: 5 droplets of cypress oil, 8 droplets rosemary, 12 drops lemon

* Massage Blend: 4 droplets rosemary and 4 droplets of thyme. 8 drops peppermint. 10 droplets grapefruit.

* Nausea Blend: 10 droplets peppermint, 30 droplets lavender

## Natural Medicine: Essential Oil Remedies

Here are some of the many ways that essential oils can be used to treat common ailments and to get you feeling better.

* Use peppermint and lavender oil to relieve migraines. Massage the temples with this oil to relieve a migraine or bad headache.

* Enhance your workout energy by inhaling peppermint oil just before exercising to help with fatigue.

* Reduces cough: Add a few drops eucalyptus oil into some hot, steamy water or your diffuser. Inhaling this oil will clear the blocked nose passages.

* Reduce fever: Place 1-3 drops each of peppermint, lavender, and eucalyptus essential oils on a dampened cloth. This liquid should be sprayed all over the body.

* Fix broken bones: Use this mixture of cypress oil, fir and helichrysum oils on the affected area to help heal broken bones.

* Arthritis relief - Combine 2 drops of lemongrass oil, cypress and wintergreen oils into a non-scented lotion. Massage directly the area where you are experiencing pain.

* Apply lavender oil directly to bites and stings.

Mix three drops of coconut and one droplet of tea tree oils together to treat ringworm. Massage the infected area directly twice per day.

* Improve digestion: Add 2 drops of ginger oil, peppermint and fennel oils together to improve digestion.

* Treat head lice by combining 3 drops each of lavender, thyme, and Eucalyptus oils. Use this mixture directly on the scalp to cure it. Place a showercap on your head and let it dry for about half an hour. Rinse your hair.

* Bronchitis and asthma treatment: Combine coconut oil, peppermint oil, and eucalyptus oil together. Massage on neck and chest.

* To heal your skin, combine 2 drops tea tree oil and 2 drops of unscented oil. To heal blistered skin, apply 5+ times per day.

*Bruise Treatment: Mix 5 drops of lavender oil and 4 ounces water. Apply to the affected area.

* For sunburn relief, combine chamomile and lavandin oils with a tablespoon each of coconut oil. Use a cotton ball to apply the oil directly onto the skin. You will see a decrease in sunburns over time.

* Concentration booster - Inhale peppermint or grapefruit oils.

* Poison oak and poison Ivy Treatment: Take 3 drops of peppermint essential oil and mix it with unscented oil. Place it on the affected area.

* Sore feet - Pour 10 drops peppermint oil and 1 tablespoon Epsom Salt into a tub of boiling water. Let the feet soak for a few minutes to reduce soreness.

* Help your metabolism by mixing cinnamon, ginger and grapefruit oils three times daily.

* Reduce teeth grinding. Massage 1-3 drops of lavender essential oil into your bottom and right behind your ears before you go to bed.

* Reduce PMS symptoms: Add 2 drops of rosemary, basil, or sage oil to a small bowl. Apply the mixture to a wet/moistened towel and place in your abdomen.

* Reduce morning nausea by adding a few drops ginger, orange and lemon oils to a damp cloth. Slowly inhale.

* Reduce food cravings by inhaling both peppermint oil and cinnamon oil. This will help to curb appetite and balance blood sugars.

* To reduce back and neck pains, mix cayenne oil, ginger, cypress and peppermint oils with coconut oil.

* For at least a week, take 3 drops of frankincense & oregano oils daily to kick a cold.

* Hangover relief - Add 6 drops of lemon and rosemary oils to warm water.

## Chapter 21: Natural Remedies - Menopause Symptoms

It can be difficult for many women to deal with menopause symptoms. Some people report experiencing hot flashes that cause major mood changes. There are people who feel the need to sweat and have chills no matter what time it is. These sensations can be experienced by women both in pre-menopause and officially in menopause.

There are many options for treating it. The best treatment is to take medication or make lifestyle changes. The problem isn't always simple and everyone isn't willing to accept medication.

You can find herbal solutions to this problem.

Soy

Soy foods have isoflavones, which aid in balancing hormone levels. It can also be used to stimulate estrogen activity. While there are many options for soy supplements, it has been shown that natural soy food is the best source of isoflavones. There are plenty of options for soy-based food including tempeh and soymilk.

## Flaxseed

This has a component called Linin that is vital for the regulation of hormone metabolism. Preparing the seeds takes very little time. Make sure to use a grinder to grind the seeds every day.

## Dong Quai

It is commonly used in China as well as the West when it comes supporting and maintaining the balance between female hormones. However, it does nothing to increase estrogenic activity. Take care not to take this herb if you are experiencing heavy bleeding during menopause.

## Black Cohosh

This product will help you to reduce the discomforts of menopause (hot flashes) It balances hormone levels and helps reduce hot flashes. There have been some reports that women are not satisfied with the results. It can be more efficient for some people than for others. The reason for this is still unknown.

## Vitamin E

Daily intakes of this herb will not only improve the skin's condition and detoxify the body but can also be used to reduce hot flashes in women going through menopause.

Evening Primrose

Most women will experience dry skin and hair loss. Evening primrose has the ability to alleviate all these symptoms. It makes it easier and more manageable.

## Chapter 22: Other Gi Tract Issues - Gas, Heartburn Irritable Bowel Stomach Ache And Ulcers

While nausea, bloating constipation diarrhea and abdominal discomfort are all common issues in issues dealing with the GI Tract (mostly), there are many other annoying and persistent GI Tract issues. The following topics will be addressed: gas, heartburns, irritable stool, stomach pain, and ulcers.

Gas

Problem: The problem is that the laundry list of what causes gas is much longer than the one at the movie theater ladies' room. There are many options, but there is a good alternative.

Perhaps your mom warned you not to "wolf" down your food. You're likely to be swallowing gas which causes you burp and passes gas. Another reason to slow down when you eat is to chew properly. Without proper chewing, you may miss important enzyme activity in the salivary glands (salivary amylase). The colon ferments partially chewed foods as they enter the stomach.

Gas is caused by fermentation. The majority of gas is caused by foods that aren't digested in your stomach and small intestine. Once that happens, it then passes into your colon in a partially digested condition.

Complex carbohydrates and foods with complex carbs might present a challenge for the digestion system. They might not be able to reach the colon completely, which could cause gas.

*Beans

*Any legume

*Cabbage

*Broccoli

*Brussels sprouts

*Cauliflower

Complex carbohydrates and complex cellulose can be found in vegetables such as the ones mentioned. This can make them difficult to digest for small intestines. These compounds are then broken down by colon bacteria. Gas is also produced.

Flatulence is also possible in fruits such apricots (raisins), prunes (prunes), and figs. They all contain fructose. Sometimes, it is not well-absorbed and the result is a colon bacteria.

These are not the only problems. Many adults, including African-Americans, lack the lactase necessary to dissolve the lactose contained in dairy products. As a result, dairy products emit gases. Carbonated drinks and foods high in fiber are also culprits. Artificial sugars, such as mannitol and xylitol, are also known to cause gas. A person can make gas and not touch food or drink because of the excess stomach acid. Your stomach can produce more acid than it needs, so your body makes bicarbonate in order to counteract the acid. This can lead to the formation of gas. Vitamin C in high amounts can also cause the body to produce excess and bicarbonate.

The Solution

If you're constantly taking Tums or Maalox or any other anti-acid that stops acid production or neutralizes it like calcium carbonate, you could be making the problem worse. You'll just produce more gas. Avoiding or limiting acid-producing foods and drinks is the best option.

This is the "do it yourself" way to eliminate gas. You should start by eliminating certain foods, and then be conscious of the results. Try removing dairy products first to see if it helps. Next, ask your doctor about the ELISA/ACT test. This tests for IgG antibodies and detects delayed food allergy reactions. These are the steps you can take to reduce gas production.

No Wolfing

Gas happens when you eat your food too fast and do not chew well enough. Allow your salivary enzymes to get the job done. Slow down.

Steam Your Veggies

Steaming vegetables softens the cellulose and makes them easier for digestion.

Fiber

Although a high fiber diet is healthy, it is not easy to digest. Your GI Tract has to adapt to this diet. In order to increase fiber in your diet gradually, you should drink plenty of water and keep hydrated.

## Beano

Beano works well with fibrous food, and is very effective in reducing gas. Beano can be taken in the morning with high-fiber cereal. Beano is a pharmacy-purchased item that contains Simethicone. Please follow the directions on your package.

## Lactose-free

Try switching to dairy products that are lactose-free or buying "lactaid," which aids with digestion of lactose.

## Miso Soup

Miso soup is made from a fermented soybean paste and is great source of fructo-oligosaccahrides (FOS). FOS encourages the growth of "friendlybacteria," which, in turn, aids in digestion. FOS is also found in artichokes and asparagus. It's also present in most fermented foods such as sauerkraut (made from soybeans), tempeh and soyabean. Increase the intake of fermented foods to reduce your gas.

Probiotics

Yogurt, which is a living culture food, contains active cultures from lactobacillus acidophilus (or lactobacillus brifidus). For active cultures, check the label (just take a probiotic supplement).

Probiotics might cause more bloating or gas initially. Take probiotics one at a time to minimize gas and bloating. It is worth trying different combinations to find the right probiotics. They can help you digest food and reduce gas.

Ginger

Ginger is great for gassiness. You can either take 200 mgs of ginger in tablet form, or you can drink ginger tea. Ginger tea is made with 2 teaspoons ginger powder (available at your local grocery store). You can use fresh ginger that has been graded for the tea. Before you enjoy, strain it.

Fennel Seeds

Fennel seeds are licorice flavored. They have 8% of volatile oil, which reduces gas and is antispasmodic. Look out for fennel seed in your supermarket's spice section. Take 1/2 teaspoon and chew it whenever you feel gassy.

Marshmallow Root & Slippery Elm

Both make excellent after-dinner beverages. Both these herbs help to soothe the stomach and coat your intestinal tract. Look for a combination of herbal teas that can aid digestion at your local heath foods store. Two tablespoons of the prepared tea should be boiled in a cup. Allow to steep for ten minutes. Then strain it and serve.

Heartburn

The Problem: Heartburn isn't related to the heart. Some of these symptoms can mimic a heart attack. Acid reflux, or heartburn, refers to irritation of the stomach caused by stomach acid.

With the help gravity, a muscle valve, the lower esophageal sphincter - or LES - keeps stomach acids inside the stomach. The LES can be found at the junction between the stomach and the esophagus. The LES is normally open to allow food to pass into your stomach. However, if the LES does not close tightly enough or is too loose, stomach acid may seep into the esophagus causing a burning sensation. Acid reflux does not cause burning sensations in the lower half of the esophagus. A burning sensation can occur when stomach acid reaches upper one-third the food tube. Patients mistakenly call it heartburn because of its proximity to the heart.

While occasional heartburn is not dangerous and is not a serious condition, persistent heartburn can be a sign of more serious issues. Heartburn is common in about 10% of Americans and 50% of pregnant woman. It's not a frequent problem for 30%.

What causes this very common problem to occur? Foods like:

*Tomato-based dishes

*Coffee (both regular, and decaf).

*Citrus fruits

*Onions

*Garlic

*Chocolate

*Wine

*Beer

All of the preceding conditions can trigger acid reflux. Other conditions can also cause burning sensations.

*Simply bend at the waist.

*Wearing tight, waistband clothes.

*Excessive abdominal weight

*Stress

Anything that causes a disruption in the function or movement of the wavelike muscles contractions (peristalsis), is harmful to the digestive system.

Many people live in stressful circumstances, overeat, or drink too much coffee. It is not surprising that heartburn medications are one of the most sought-after drugs on the globe.

Some side-effects are possible with the use of antibiotics.

*Famotidine, also known as Pepcid, is an acid reducer that can cause headaches, constipation, or even diarrhea.

*Ranitidine (CVS), an acid reducer, may cause all of these.

*Cimetodine or Tagamet, an acid reducer that can cause lightheadedness/dizziness, may be used.

*Omeprazole Magnesium OTC acid decreaser can cause light headedness or sweating.

*Lansoprazole (Prevacid), Proton-pump inhibitor. Stops acid production within 24 hours. Prevacid and Proton-pump inhibitors like Prevacid have a problem. Your stomach then produces more acid, which can lead to more heartburn.

The above antacid list is not complete. There are far too many antacids for me to list. Each antacid comes with the following warning: Stop using them if you have heartburn for more than a few hours.

The market for antacids has a multi-billion-dollar market. However, there are many natural remedies available that will help you avoid this trap.

The Solution

A better way to avoid the dangers of over-using the antacids is to minimize the number of triggers.

*Reduce your coffee consumption

*Get rid of tight clothes (jeans).

*Eat smaller meals

Avoid foods such as tomato dishes, hot salsas, wine, and beer

*Avoid stress

*Avoid late night meals

If you are experiencing chest pains, do not hesitate to visit the emergency department.

But let's be positive and say your burning sensation in the chest is simple heartburn...fortunately, there are numerous natural remedies that don't involve pharmaceuticals:

Aloe Vera

The acid reflux can be quickly relieved with the help of the succulent desert plant juice. It does this by coating the stomach with a mucus like coating, and keeping the stomach acid right where it belongs (in your stomach).

Turmeric

Turmeric, the spice that gives curry its distinct flavor, helps break down fats, which can lead too heartburn. Turmeric can be bought in capsules at your local HFS.

Slippery Elm

Your saliva and this herb interact to form a mucous like coating as it moves down the esophagus. It absorbs acids from the stomach as well as the food tube. Mix 1 teaspoon of slippery alm bark (available at your local HFS), in 1/2 cup boiling water. Allow it to cool, then make a tea and enjoy it two to four times daily.

Papaya

A cup of papaya juice with 1 teaspoon of sugar and two pitches each of cardamom will help to ease acid reflux.

Lemon Aid

Melissa or lemon balm can be used to soothe heartburn and relax your nerves. In a large pot, boil the leaves. Allow the water to simmer for 10 minutes. After that, strain the tea. You can do this up to three more times per day.

Gentian Root Tincture

Gentian, a bitter herb with powerful medicinal properties, will boost your saliva, enzyme production, and stimulate digestion. It will relieve heartburn from after-meal. You can add 1 teaspoon of gentianroot tincture to one cup of water. Take it out 15 minutes before you start eating. Your local HFS can provide Gentian root extract.

Licorice

If you enjoy licorice you're in luck. You can take two 380mg tablets deglycyrrhizinated or DGL licorice 20 minutes before you eat. It will calm acid backup and help with indigestion. It may also soothe an inflamed esophagus.

Habits

Our habits dictate "how" and "what" we do. Here are some habits to help prevent acid reflux from happening:

*Eat dinner three hours prior to bedtime

*Take a relaxing stroll after you finish your meal (between 10 and 15 minutes).

*When you retire, lay down on a wedge shaped pillow that will raise your entire torso. Avoid stacking heavy pillows under your head. That can lead to a compressed stomach.

*Lie on your left side. This will lower the stomach/esophagus, which inhibits acid reflux.

Irritable Bowel

Problem: There are many diseases associated with central GI Tract disorders, including depression, migraines and sinusitis. These diseases have been linked to specific patterns and responses to food allergies. All of these diseases can be linked to Irritable Bowel Syndrome.

If you have had symptoms of irritable intestinal syndrome for more than three months, including mucus in your stool, gas, sudden urgency or straining, then you may be suffering from hypersensitive digestion tract. This means that your colon can spasm at the slightest irritation caused by foods you are allergic to or intolerable to.

*Coffee

*Tea

*Chocolate

IBS is most common during periods and hormone imbalances. IBS can also be triggered by emotional problems. Emotional upsets can trigger IBS. The spasms may cause the colon content to shift too slowly (constipation), and too quickly (diarrhea). IBS patients are also hypersensitive. Even normal contractions caused by digesting food can result in intense pain.

The Solution

Although antispasmodic medicines may be an option, there are significant side effects, including blurred vision and dry lips. IBS sufferers often get relief without having to resort to medication.

Food triggers

Research has shown that IBS patients are almost three quarters likely to be allergic or intolerance to at most one or two foods. A quarter of people with IBS report that they have experienced relief by keeping a food log. A food diary can help you identify and eliminate the problematic foods from your diet. Examples:

*Reduce allergens by cooking raw vegetables

*Eat smaller portions to reduce intestinal load

*Wheat (allergic for gluten)

*Dairy Products - Allergic to Lactose

*Sweeteners: sorbitol orxylitol

*Coffee (caffeine response)

Artichoke Leaf Extract

In one study, IBS sufferers who used capsules of artichoke leaves extract twice daily for six week were found to have significantly reduced their cramps and constipation. The liquid and capsule versions of artichoke Leaf Extract are both available at your local HFS.

Fennel

Fennel can be described as having a licorice taste. Fennel tea has antispasmodic properties and can reduce gastric and intestinal bloating. It is one of your best defenses against IBS. Boil 1 teaspoon of fennel, and 1 slice of fresh Ginger in a cup. Allow it to steep for 5-10 mins, then strain the mixture and serve. Do this three times per day. You can also chew the fennel seed.

## Peppermint

Peppermint's refreshing aroma and flavor is remarkable. This herb aids digestion and has antispasmodic characteristics. It is also known to help fight yeast growth in the GI Tract. This can result in gas formation and bloating which can cause severe pain. Take three to five capsules of enteric -coated peppermint essential oil daily. At your local HFS.

## Roast or Steam

It is possible to remove raw vegetables from IBS patients' diets by steaming or roasting your vegetables. The cellulose becomes easier to digest through cooking, which reduces gas formation.

## Rice

Rice can reduce diarrhea, protect the mucous liner of the GI tract, reduce IBS and help with IBS. You should not cook one cup of rice with only two cups of liquid. Instead, use four cups. After the normal cooking cycle is completed, drain the extra water. Then add some sugar to taste and enjoy it throughout your day. Try rice bran extract capsules...100mgs three times daily. It acts like rice water.

## Psyllium

IBS can be helped by fiber. Psyllium can be described as a powdered, water-soluble fiber. To each glass of water add a heaping teaspoon of powder every morning. Stir the mixture and then drink the whole glass. Next, drink another glass. 8-10 glasses of water are recommended daily.

## Stomach Ache

The Problem: The main cause of stomachache is overindulgence, which is linked with indigestion. Overindulgence is a sign that the stomach produces more stomach acid. Excessive stomach acid can cause discomfort, especially if it is released through the cardiac sphincter. This acid can then cause a burning sensation and damage to the esophagus.

Another way to get stomach cramps is to "gobble" or "wolf" your food. Hurriedly swallowing food results in very little enzyme action from saliva (saliva is a source of an enzyme called amylase which breaks down carbohydrates). It takes saliva very little time to perform its task, so it is important to swallow your food quickly. Stomach acid will block the enzyme from working. This means digestion is left up to the GI system intestine. This creates bacterial fermentation and gas.

Eating certain gas-producing foods such as:

*Beans

*Cauliflower

*Dairy Products (if intolerant to lactose)

## Chapter 23: Looking Ten Years Younger And Feeling Good About It!

After you have completed 9 chapters, you will be excited to go through the rest of the book. This is the best way to live a happier, healthier life.

All of the knowledge you have gained so far should be taken into consideration. It's not enough to just jump in and know everything. Here are the last considerations before making any changes in your beauty regime:

* Health concerns/issues

Consider your current health status before making any changes to your diet. Your health should be considered when making changes to your diet and lifestyle. You don't want to get sick from it.

You should always seek advice from your doctor before making any changes to your health, especially if you have a sensitive condition such as. pregnant, lactating, etc. This will give your peace of mind.

* Allergic triggers

Common misconception is that skin irritations can't occur if they are natural. This is completely incorrect! It is possible for anyone to experience allergic reactions, no matter what the product's purity or naturalness. For instance, some people are naturally allergic milk (lactose sensitive), mint, or shrimp. This means you need to be familiar with the ingredients of what you're putting into your body, as well as your allergy triggers. Honey and coconut oil can be allergenic so you should stop using them if you have an allergy. There are other products that can be used on your skin, which is the good news. All you have to do is find the right one for you.

* Time and budget

Also, budget and time should be considered. You will often find that natural products can be more difficult to locate than commercial products. You will find it worth it in the long run!

* Positive mindset

The last but not least, it is important to have the right mindset. Being beautiful and young does not necessarily mean looking younger. Sometimes you don't need to look good to feel happy. Be sure to do the things you enjoy and not because of what others think. It's your life, so you have to make the effort and reap what it brings.

You are now prepared to take a step 10 years younger than yourself! Discover all that life has to give you and feel more energetic, healthy, and younger.

## Chapter 24: Bronchitis, Coughs, And Chest Infections

Simply put, chest infection refers to an illness that affects your lungs. Bronchitis occurs when the infection affects the large airways. In the case of the smaller air sacs, it's called pneumonia. These infections are very common in the elderly.

Chest infections are common in spring and winter. They can be sudden or gradual.

Common symptoms are difficulty breathing, coughing green or brown colored phlegms, headaches and fever.

Chest infection can be serious. The following chapters contain remedies that can be used to treat symptoms. However, professional treatment is advised.

REMEDIES

For bronchitis or coughs, slice a Spanish onions and place the slices in an oval-shaped bowl. The basin should be covered tightly and left to rest for twelve hours. After 12 hours, the juice should be extracted from the basin. Make a syrup by combining the juice from crushed strawberries and cane sugar.

To relieve symptoms, take one teaspoonful each of the syrups.

The use of hot lemon juice to relieve congestion is also recommended.

Turnip juice, boiling with sugar, is an ancient remedy for chronic bronchitis. It is important to grate the turnips, then squeeze out the juice. 2 1/2 oz. The mixture is boiled until slightly thickened. It can be taken up to three times daily.

One or two English onions can be placed in a bag of muslin and pounded to a pulp to make an excellent poultice. The chest should be cleaned and the poultice renewed every three to four hours.

BRUISES

Bruises refer to skin imperfections caused by blood trapped underneath the skin's surface. They develop when blood vessels known by capillaries become damaged and the skin is not broken.

Not only is it unsightly but can also cause pain, especially when there is swelling. They often start as a small red mark and then become more severe over time. They often disappear but can sometimes remain dark after they heal.

REMEDIES

Plaster of banana skin can be applied to inflamed, sprained or bruised areas.

RHEUMATISM

Rheumatism, which is used in general to describe a range joint, connective tissue, and muscle pain symptoms.

It is most commonly caused by inflammation. The intensity of the pain varies. Sometimes, this pain can also be associated with stiff joints or limited movement.

REMEDIES

Celery is good for relieving the symptoms associated with rheumatism.

The following foods are believed to aid in the treatment of rheumatism: asparagus, strawberries, lemons.

An external remedy that is used to treat rheumatism is to use a strained liquid made from 1lb of potatoes. The liquid is then boiled in 2pints (water) until it reduces in volume to 1 liter.

SORE THE THROAT

A sore sore throat is a condition where there are symptoms like irritation, difficulty speaking, discomfort, or pain when eating. It can also affect speech.

Sore throats can result from colds, influenza, or laryngitis. Another cause is pollution, smoking and a dry environment.

REMEDIES

Blackcurrant is one of the most effective remedies for sore throats. You can make it by heating half a pint and then adding one tablespoonful of blackcurrant jelly/ja to the boiling water.

Another traditional way to treat a sore is taking a raw ripe fruit and slicing it into a fine pulp using a teaspoon. This pulp can be taken by the spoonful and held against your throat for as long time as possible.

For sore throats, it is also soothing to use the pineapple.

STINGS, BITES and the like

Most common stings/bites are caused by insects or bugs. They inject venom, or another substance into the skin. These are typically mild and include a slight swelling, reddening, mild stinging, and itching.

Reaction to stings and bites will depend on the individual skin reaction as well the type of the venom. Some people will experience an allergic reaction to foreign substances. A victim who is not treated immediately after the sting or bite could develop allergic reactions, such as hives or fever.

While some bugs and insects are extremely poisonous, it is very rare. You may experience nausea, abdominal pains, difficulty breathing, and facial swelling. These advanced symptoms are easily treated with quick intervention.

It is best to get rid of any stings that are embedded in the skin. To prevent more severe reactions, it is important to treat the affected area with an appropriate remedy.

## REMEDIES

Raw onions are an effective antiseptic. Apply them to the affected areas.

## Chapter 25: Other Tips To Get Ridof Hypertension

Power Walks

Research has shown that patients suffering from hypertension who exercised at a steady pace were able to lower their blood pressure by as much as 8 mmhg. This is in comparison with 6 mmhg. Because exercise improves the efficiency of oxygen use, this can be explained by studies. This means the heart doesn't have as much to pump the blood. Most experts recommend at least 30 mins of vigorous cardio each day. Your heart should be challenged by your ability to increase the distance and speed of your power walking.

Potassium should be a top priority

To lower blood pressure, it is essential to eat potassium-rich vegetables. Experts suggest that you consume between 2000 and 4,000 mg per day. Sweet potatoes, sweet potatoes potatoes, kidney beans, kidney beans, tomato juice, cantaloupe and bananas are all potassium-rich food options.

Reduce Your Salt Intake

Although some people are more prone to hypertension due to their sodium (or salt) sensitivities, all people with hypertension should cut down on salt intake. Most experts recommend that we consume no more than 1,500 mg of sodium daily. This is less than the daily intake of Americans on average. One teaspoon of salt contains about 1,200mg sodium. It is important to reduce salt intake and to replace salt with herbs, lemons, spices or salt-free seasoning mixtures.

Dark Chocolate is the Best!

Dark chocolate is sweet when you need it. Flavanols are found in dark chocolate, which can make blood vessels more elastic. One study showed that 18 percent patients who ate dark chocolat every day experienced a decrease of their blood pressure. Experts suggest consuming 1/2 ounces dark chocolate that contains at most 70-percent cocoa in order to lower blood pressure.

A little alcohol is okay

Drinking too much alcohol is not good for your health. However, it can actually lower blood pressure than drinking no alcohol. However, this doesn't mean that you should drink to your heart's content every night. Limiting your intake to 1 drink (e.g., 5 ounces wine, 12 beer, or 1.5-ounces spirits) is the best thing. Keep in mind that moderate alcohol can be good for your heart. But, too much of it can do more harm that good.

Switch to decaf

While there are many theories on the effect of caffeine in blood pressure that have been discussed for years, a Duke University Medical Center research found that drinking 500mg of caffeine, which equals three 8-ounce cups, increases blood pressure by around 4 mmhg. You can feel the effects even after you go to sleep.

Work Less

If you work over 41 hours per week, your chances of getting hypertension increase by 15%. Overworking increases your stress levels and makes it difficult to eat healthy food and get enough exercise.

Relax and Listen to Music

Music can be a relaxing way to lower blood pressure. You don't have to listen to the same music every day. Research has shown that listening for 30 minutes to classical, Celtic, or Indian music a day can have a profound impact on your blood pressure.

Snoring should be checked out

Obstructive sleeping apnea can be diagnosed by your ability to snore. University of Alabama research found that people suffering from sleep apnea had higher levels of the hormone aldosterone. Aldosterone is a hormone which raises blood pressure. Experts have even estimated that 50% of sleep apnea sufferers also have high blood pressure.

Eat More Soy

The Journal of the American Heart Associated published a study that found that replacing refined carbohydrates in diets that are high in soy protein or milk protein can help lower blood pressure in hypertension patients.

# Chapter 26: Reiki

A brief overview of Reiki and its alternative healing power.

Reiki is a method to heal, self-heal, and distance heal. It involves gently placing your hands on a person or object (e.g. a photograph).

This healing method was discovered in Japan by Mikao Usui (1865 – 1926), a Japanese Buddhist.

It is becoming more popular and nurses in some countries are being trained to practice Reiki on patients in hospitals.

Reiki Explained

Reiki is noninvasive and is performed by a Reiki practitioner (or master) (the difference is that a master can teach it while a practitioner only practices it).

Energy is everywhere. Reiki practitioners have their "bungs," which allow energy to flow freely, and thus are able to access the energy channel. This allows energy to flow through them, and the principle behind Reiki is that they are "conductors". They act as conductors of energy and are unaffected by the mood or humor of patients. The Reiki practitioner's thoughts or feelings do not affect the patient.

Reiki, also pronounced "raykey" (laykey in Japan) can be described as two words. Rei is roughly the wisdom of nature, while Ki is the "lifeform energy". Ki flows through people and animals as well as plants and non-living objects.

Electromagnetic energy can be described as both an energy field that surrounds or touches us and a part our bodies. This is what most people call the "aura", although some people refer to it as "vibes" because it is indeed an energy field that vibrates.

Reiki helps to heal and repair the energy fields that can be damaged. It can help you feel better, even if you're ill.

Reiki benefits

How Reiki works for you depends on the problems you are facing. Each person is unique. Here are some things Reiki can do:

Boosts the body's ability to self heal

Aids to Sleep

Chronic problems such as asthma, eczema etc. can be treated

Headaches - a quick Reiki treatment can make a headache disappear

This program helps you break your addictions

Immune system improvement

Lower your blood pressure

Reiki can be used to reduce physical injury or pain. It also promotes healing.

The body can heal itself by reducing stress

It reduces side effects associated with some therapies and drugs, such as chemotherapy

You can get rid of anxiety. This will make you feel calmer and more able to deal with your daily activities.

Toxins and Reiki help to eliminate toxins from the body

Reiki Evolution and Origin

Mikao Usui taught Reiki Ryoho Gakkai (or Usui Reiki Ryoho Gakkai) to his students. Before he died, Dr. Chujiro Hayashi was the only Japanese man who could teach him. The man taught Japanese people to be Reiki practitioners, but at first, he was unable to give it to anyone.

Hawayo Takata saw a Japanese lady named Hawayo Takata in his clinic in 1935. She was cured of a cancerous tumor by him and begged him to teach them how to help others. He accepted her request and taught her how Reiki practitioners work. Two years later she went back to Hawaii to open a Reiki center. Hayashi visited her in 1938 and taught her level three, so she could also be a teacher.

There are two possible explanations.

One person claims that all Japanese Reiki practitioners were killed by the war. Ms Takata is the only person who can train more teachers.

Another explanation is that the Gakkai's Reiki Society has been so secretive and closed, that no one can know what happens, who is there, or what they do. (The American government after WWII banned Japanese healing techniques and ordered that only Western medicine was used.

The reason for the secrecy of the Gakkai Reiki Society is that it had to be kept secret.

However, the Hawaiian lady was able train twenty-two Reiki teachers. It is evident that she is the reason Reiki is now widely available.

This method is accepted today for healing, regardless of whether it was the original version or has been modified slightly to suit Western tastes.

Reiki is a method of healing.

There are seven major points known as "Chakras", and approximately twenty-five minor ones. Chakras refer to a spiral of energy that is located along the spine. Energy radiates from this area through Chakras.

This is a listing of all the major Chakras. It also includes a few examples of how each Chakra's energy can be used for.

The principal Chakras are:

* 1st the base the spine -legs. bones. feet. Immune system

* 2nd naval – sexual organs (benthic, bladder, appendix), large intestines, lower vertebraes, pelvis, and hips

* 3rd solar Plxus – middle spine, abdomen and stomach, upper intestines and internal organs (liver. kidneys. gall bladder. pancreas.

* 4th/mid chest - heart and circulation. Shoulders, arms, heart and breathing. Ribs/breasts. diaphragm.

* 5th throat –, thyroid, trachea and neck vertebrae. Mouth, teeth and gums.

* 6th brow: Brain, nervous systems, eyes, ears, nose and brain

* 7th crown - skin, muscle and skeletal system

Chakras are a vital part the body's energy. They are also where Reiki healing is possible.

The patient is either able to lay down on a massage table, or he can sit in a comfortable chair. No need to take off clothing. Shoes are not required.

The energy flows from the therapist's hands as they lightly touch the Chakra points. The energy is "intelligent", meaning it will naturally go to the places it needs to heal, even if it's not where you wanted.

Some sensations or feelings can be felt by the practitioner or patient. They include tingling sensations, hot or cool sensations, and tingling sensations.

Some patients experience a deep sleep during treatment. These are all manifestations of energy being released.

Reiki Levels

There are three levels for Reiki.

First level: The practitioner's channels are open and will remain open throughout his entire life.

Second level: The channels are open more to allow distance healing

Third level - This is when the practitioner can become a master teacher and can also teach Reiki to others

It's interesting to note, however, that Reiki energy is not visible by the human eyes, but can be picked up using a Kirlian Camera. Semyon Kirlian found out accidentally that an image can be produced by touching a photographic plate. Contact photography became a term for this phenomenon.

One important point is that Reiki should not ever be used on fractured bones. It may speed up the healing process, causing the bone to become too hard or weaker.

A personal note: My partner, a Reiki practitioner, has performed Reiki on several people who fell asleep, left their homes limping, left running, and came back feeling sad and depressed.

He performs Reiki to me when I have migraines. Unfortunately, this does not always work. However, it will often lessen the attack and decrease the time it takes to last from three days to one-and-a-half days.

If done properly, the process is noninvasive and can make you look great.

This article should not be interpreted as a substitute for expert medical advice. You should consult your physician before taking any steps to improve your health.

Vinegar

A history of vinegar including the uses and nutritional information.

Vinegar and its history

Because it is so old, there are no records of where vinegar was found.

It has been mentioned by ancient Egyptians (Greeks), Chinese and the Bible.

Vinegar is usually made by letting alcohol react with air. It can be produced by any fruit, vegetable, or grain that is suitable to make alcohol.

In the olden days, people were known to try anything and waste nothing. Therefore, it is presumed that this liquid was accidentally made by someone who tried to use it.

"Medicine men", who had no formal training, used to travel across the country selling miracle drugs and magic potion. They claimed that these potions could cure any condition and could also be used for other purposes. Today, this idea is ridiculed. But if they were selling vinegar, they might have been right in many instances.

Vinegar is used as a disinfectant. It is an anti-bacterial agent that cleans and preserves food. Evidence has been found to support this claim in 2030 BCE. The Babylonians claimed to have discovered these properties in 5000 BCE. However there is no definitive evidence.

Vinegar: A Wine for All Ages

Cleopatra believed in vinegar as a key component of a beauty treatment. Hippocrates (4000 BCE), established vinegar's use as an internal and external medication, as well as as as an antibiotic.

It has been used around the globe to prevent blood clots and as an anti-inflammatory. Also, it is used for headaches, burns, and elimination of toxins.

Vinegar was used for disinfection in Bubonic Plague outbreaks. It was also used by ships (including Christopher Columbus's Nina Pinta and Santa Maria) to wipe the decks.

Another use of the sand was by Hannibal, who used it as a way to get rid of boulders while crossing the Alps. Cleopatra, on the other hand, used it to dissolve pearls in order to eat them.

Vinegar Types and Their Uses

There are many types of them, but these are the main ones.

Apple Cider Vinegar

Hippocrates loved it and used as an antibiotic. It kills bacteria, decreases inflammation, and disinfects. The

Many people report that it helped them lose weight, reduce the symptoms of arthritis and even cure dandruff. Others have claimed it helped with diabetes and osteoporosis.

It reduces calcium excretion and helps circulation.

For many, a glass of Apple Cider Vinegar diluted daily (about one part vinegar to six parts water) has been proven to lower cholesterol. It has been shown to lower cholesterol in animals, but not enough research with humans to confirm this. (This is not surprising as there are few studies that have been done on natural medicine.

It is known for its extraordinary curative powers and is called the "King Vinegars". The number of nutrients in this liquid is staggering (and these are just some).

Potassium, Calcium, Magnesium, Phosphorus, Copper, Iron, Silicone, Pectin, Vitamins; A, B1, B2, B6, C, E, Beta-carotene

This is used for pickling. It has a milder flavour than other types of vinegar.

Apple Cider Vinegar is a good choice for preserving cooked fruits, or adding spices to them.

Balsamic

This ancient artifact is approximately 1,000 years old and comes from Modena Italy.

This is an excellent way to caramelize vegetables. It is healthier than sugar and is also less sweet. It is great for marinades, and it can also be used to dress salads.

Distilled Vinegar

This has a clearer or "whiter" taste and a sharper flavor than the other types. It is easy to make and cheaper to buy. This can be used to clean floors, windows, and other surfaces. It disinfects while cleaning and is much healthier than chemical household cleaners.

It is great for pickling food with strong flavors, such as garlic or onions.

It can be used to remove most types glues without the use of a chemical solvent.

This will take bad odors out of your fridge and home. Put a small cup of water in the affected area, and leave it there for several hours.

Malt Vinegar

This vinegar is darker in color and is not as tart as the other types. It has a strong, malty taste that can be used in pickling. However it can be used to pickle nuts.

The best way to get rid of bad breath is to swish some malt vinegar around the mouth after eating strong foods like onions.

Some prefer to add this type of cheese to chips or fries. Others make Pavlova with it.

Add one teaspoon of Malt Vinegar to a glass of warm water. Use this mixture to rub your hair for 20-30 mins. Your hair will look shiny and clean longer. Rinse the hair well to remove any vinegar smell.

Rice Vinegar

The Chinese introduced this dish to Japan in the fourth-century.

This can be used in sweet and sour dishes as well as stir fries.

It is often mistaken for Rice Wine Vinegar. Rice wine vinegar is vinegar that has rice wine added.

Wine Vinegar

Red Wine Vinegar makes a great pickling agent when you're adding spices. It adds body and depth to your flavour.

For making your own flavoured vinaigrette, white wine vinegar can be used as a base. You can use almost any herb or vegetable you like, but these include basil, chilli and rosemary, fennel, garlic, fruit such as banana, strawberry, pineapple, orange, and even cranberry.

To release the flavour, it is necessary to "bruise" the fruit by first lightly crushing or pounding.

You can simmer the vinegar for a few minutes to bring out the flavor of the herbs. After that, pour the vinegar over the herbs. Let cool down, seal the container and allow it to stand for up to a week before using.

This article should not be interpreted as a substitute for expert medical advice. You should consult your physician before taking any steps to improve your health.

## Chapter 27: Insomnia Causes And Symptoms

It is important to identify the root cause if you suffer from insomnia. Half of insomnia cases are due to stress, depression and anxiety. The environment in which you sleep, your health and your daily habits all can contribute to sleepless nights. It is important to identify all the possible causes and then take the necessary steps to correct the situation. Once you know the cause, you can determine the correct treatment.

To find the best way to solve your sleep problems you'll need to become a great sleep detective. Begin by getting a brand new notebook. Make it your'sleep diary'. You can use the first pages of the notebook for investigating the reason behind your insomnia. These pages will help you to determine if you're experiencing stress or have just experienced an emotional or mental-disturbing experience. If so, take down specific details of the root cause of your stress. Also, note your reaction to it.

# Conclusion

While herbs can be beneficial for optimal health, make sure to check with your physician before you use them. It is important to seek advice from your doctor before you use herbs, especially if you are pregnant. This is also true for diabetics. Some active ingredients could cause allergies. It is important to remember that herbal medicine should be beneficial for your health, rather than causing more problems.